Nutrition Handbook
for
Community Workers
in the Tropics

Second edition

Caribbean Food and Nutrition Institute (PAHO/WHO)
in collaboration with
Ministry of Health, Jamaica

in co-operation with
Caribbean Food and Nutrition Institute

MACMILLAN

Macmillan Education
Between Towns Road, Oxford OX4 3PP
A division of Macmillan Publishers Limited
Companies and representatives throughout the world

ISBN 0333 57755 8

First CFNI edition published 1982

First international edition 1986

This edition 1993

www.macmillan-africa.com

Published in conjunction with Teaching Aids at Low Costs, PO Box 49,
St Albans, Herts AL1 4AX, England. TALC received assistance in the
production of this book at a low cost edition from the Swedish
International Development Authority.

Cover hotograph courtesy of John and Penny Hubley

Printed and bound in Malaysia

2007 2006 2005 2004 2003
14 13 12 11 10 9 8

PREFACE

I. HOW THE HANDBOOK WAS DEVELOPED

When the World Health Organization first published its 'Manual on Nutrition Training for Community Health Workers', different countries were asked to try it out and see how they could use it.

Jamaica was one of the countries in which the manual was tested. This was done by the Ministry of Health, working along with the Caribbean Food and Nutrition Institute (CFNI).

The Ministry of Health and CFNI found that they could use the manual, but they felt that they would prefer to use one written specifically for their part of the world. They also believed that all community workers, not only health workers, could use the manual on food and nutrition in their work.

The Ministry of Health and CFNI then decided to write their own Handbook of which this is the third edition.

The first edition of the Handbook was tested by community health aides and other community workers in Jamaica and other Caribbean countries. It was then reviewed by CFNI, PAHO and FAO staff members, corrected and printed. After being used for a number of years, a second edition was prepared with the support of the WHO/UNICEF Joint Nutrition Support Programme (JNSP) and used extensively in all member countries, particularly Dominica and St. Vincent and the Grenadines. It was also used as a text for the Community Nutrition course conducted through the University of the West Indies Distance Teaching facility (UWIDITE) which links several member countries.

In 1986 an international edition was jointly published by Macmillan Publishers and CFNI, with help from, TALC and SIDA. Slight changes were made to the text to make it more broadly relevant to the tropics, especially in the kinds of food mentioned.

This second international edition was published in 1993 with help from TALC.

II. WHO CAN USE THIS BOOK?

This Handbook has been written to help community workers in different government and non-government agencies, institutions or sectors, who are working together for the development of their country. Some of these sectors are health, food and nutrition, agriculture, community development and education, also non-government organizations (NGOs). Each of these sectors has its own special responsibilities in the running of a country, and the workers in each sector need certain kinds of information to help them do their jobs properly.

Most of the information in this Handbook will be more useful for people who work in the health, food and nutrition sectors than in others. However, we strongly urge you to read every chapter of the Handbook for your own personal enrichment, even though you may not necessarily use all the information in your daily work.

III. WHAT THE HANDBOOK IS ABOUT

This 'Nutrition Handbook for Community Workers' shows that the causes of food and nutrition problems are many and varied and involve several different sectors. So to solve these problems, dedication is needed from workers attached to different sectors who join their efforts to improve people's welfare.

It contains important information about food, nutrition, health and related subjects which will be useful in the day-to-day work of community workers from different sectors of a country. Some of the topics are:
— find out about the food and nutrition situation in the community;
— working with people in the community;
— selecting, storing and using foods carefully;
— nutrition for pregnant and breastfeeding women;
— malnutrition;
— Diarrhoea, obesity, diabetes and high blood pressure.

IV. HOW THE HANDBOOK IS ORGANIZED

The Handbook is made up of two parts: Chapters and Annexes.

The chapters
The chapters contain information on different health, food and nutrition subjects. Each chapter starts by telling you what you should be able to do when you have finished studying the chapter. You can make best use of the Handbook if you consider carefully if this is what you expect to get.

If you want to know and be able to do more than the chapter sets out to do, you may need to add to the information it contains. In the

Annexes is a list of other sources of information. These are books and other resources which will give you more detailed information about the topics in which you are most interested.

When you read the chapter you will notice that it has a number of different sections, each with its own heading, which tells exactly what that section is about. This will help you to pick out the most important facts first, then learn the others later as you need them.

All the chapters, except the first four, end with a section giving ideas and suggestions on how to teach people about what you have learned.

Chapter 1: 'Introduction'; Chapter 2: 'Working with the Community'; Chapter 3: 'Planning Food and Nutrition Education Programmes' and Chapter 4: 'Some Techniques of Good Communication', do not have this section. The purpose of these chapters is to help you develop useful skills for dealing with people and to prepare you to teach the information found in the other chapters. These chapters end with summaries of the information which has gone before. You can consult the summaries quickly if you need to refresh your memory on what to do in certain situations.

The annexes
Some of the annexes contain extra information on topics which have not been included in the book, but about which you ought to know something. The annexes will help you understand more about what you read in the chapters. You should consult these annexes often.

V. HOW TO USE THE HANDBOOK

To help you find the chapters which will be most relevant to your work in the community, here is a simple guide.

On the title page of each chapter is written the name of the chapter and a breakdown of the information it contains. At the bottom of the page you will see listsed subjects such as Health, Food and Nutrition, Agriculture, Education, Community Development; and General.

When you see these subjects you will know whether the chapter contains information on health, nutrition, agriculture, education or community development, or information which is of general interest.

We hope that you will enjoy studying this Handbook and pass on the knowledge you have gained to others in the community.

A.W. PATTERSON
Director, CFNI

ACKNOWLEDGEMENTS

Many people worked very hard to get this book written and published. Some of these people are:
— Versada Campbell, Nutrition Educator, CFNI
— Elizabeth Grant, former Nutritionist, Ministry of Health, Jamaica.
— Michal Gurney, former Director, CFNI
— Andrea Okwesa, Communication Specialist, CFNI
— Joan Peters, former Nutrition Educator, CFNI
— Winsome Williams and the staff of the Printing Unit of CFNI.

Beverley McFarlane, an artist from the Ministry of Education, Jamaica, who drew most of the pictures.

The drawing on page 143 is adapted from a graphic by Duncan Mil, The Observer London.

Other drawings were done by Colin White of the Scientific Research Council, Jamaica, and Don Miller of the School of Printing, University of the West Indies.

Professor David Morley, Tropical Child Health Unit, Unit of Child Health, University of London, provided growth and health charts in use in Africa and provided information on appropriate books and aids available from TALC.

The Handbook was field-tested in communities throughout the Caribbean. Public health nurses, medical officers, nutritionists, school teachers, nutrition assistants and community health aides are some of the people who took part in this field-test. We would like to thank them for trying out the Handbook in their programmes.

While the Handbook was being prepared some excellent suggestions were made people working in the following international organizations:
— The Pan American Health Organization (PAHO)
— The World Health Organization (WHO)
— The Food and Agriculture Organization (FAO)
— The United Nations Children's Fund (UNICEF)

Special thanks must also be given to staff members at CFNI and to Miss Norah Gibson, FAO Nutritionist who made many useful comments, and provided encouragement.

The writers of the book would like to say 'thank you' to all those who helped in one way of another. You can also help by studying and using the Handbook and then telling us what you think of it, and how it could be improved.

CONTENTS

Children who are likely to become
malnourished
Children needing special help
Preventing malnutrition
— some messages for mothers
Anaemia in young children
Ideas and suggestions for learning about
malnutrition in young children

QUALITIES A COMMUNITY WORKER SHOULD HAVE

1. Good communication skills: ability to listen, and to speak, write, or give ideas and information in any other way.

2. Respect for the ways of life, customs, traditions and beliefs of people in the community.

3. Willingness to understand people's problems and help them reach solutions through their own efforts.

(Adapted from Education for Health, Geneva, World Health Organization, 1984)

1

Introduction

Learning about the community

Identifying and solving problems

Evaluation

Summary

Food and Nutrition
Agriculture
Community Development
Education
General

WHAT YOU SHOULD BE ABLE TO DO AFTER STUDYING THIS CHAPTER

This chapter will show how to:
— identify sources of information about the community,
— identify those factors which affect the food and nutrition situation of the community,
— help the community recognize its chief food and nutrition problems, and
— help the community learn how to solve problems.

LEARNING ABOUT THE COMMUNITY

Most communities have many problems which members do not believe can be solved by them. For example, community members often see infectious diseases, sickly children and a poor water supply as problems which they cannot solve. Before problems can be solved, people in the community must first understand all the factors involved. This will help them to decide what are the best actions to take to solve their problems.

To help community members recognize, understand and deal with problems, the community worker should work with them in following some simple steps.
1. Identify food and nutrition problems in the community.
2. Decide on the chief problem.
3. Suggest causes for the problem.
4. Decide on what changes are needed to solve the problem.
5. Discuss some solutions to the problem.
6. Decide on one solution.
7. Develop a plan of action.
8. Carry out the plan.
9. Evaluate what has been done.

Use this step-by-step approach to deal with each problem that you find.

Remember, the community must take part in all these steps.

Collecting information

In order to get information on community problems, you will need to learn all about the community. You will want to know things like what people do for a living; the conditions under which they live; their backgrounds; concerns; interests, customs and traditions; way of life; what they think is rewarding or good in life; what their position is in the community; how much they know about what you want to talk about;

what they think of the work you are doing and what they think of you. You also need to know what are the common diseases in the community, and all the factors which cause food, nutrition and health problems to occur. Some of these factors are:

— *Educational*: do the people know about foods and nutrition, child care, hygiene and sanitation, etc.?
— *Social*: are living conditions overcrowded and insanitary, are mothers and children overburdened with work in the field and at home?
— *Economic*: do the farmers earn enough from selling their crops so that they can buy fertilizers and equipment, as well as support their families?
— *Cultural*: are there traditions or religious beliefs which affect diet, attitudes towards practices such as child spacing and so on?
— *Agricultural*: what kinds of food can be grown?
— *Health*: is the drinking water safe? What types of illnesses are common? Is there malnutrition? Who is malnourished? How severe is the malnutrition? Why does malnutrition occur?

This is not a full list of all the factors involved. You may not be able to collect detailed information on all these items. Information on these topics is always available from people within the community, other community workers and various government departments. The following chart shows some common topics and likely sources of information.

Food and nutrition topic	Possible sources of information
1. Nutrition and health problems: — prevalence of malnutrition; diarrhoeal diseases; anaemia; obesity; diabetes; parasitic infestations; hypertension.	Local clinic; hospital, local health workers
2. How people make their living: — main occupations; types of housing; social customs; water and sanitation.	Local leaders; people in the community
3. Community organization: — local committees (e.g. agriculture; health); farmer's groups; women's groups and other organizations.	Local leaders; other community workers

Food and nutrition topic	Possible sources of information
4. Public services: — kinds of roads; distances to schools, markets, health centres/clinics/hospital; agricultural centre; number and kinds of community workers; electricity; water; telephone.	Other community workers; Roads and Works or Public Works Department; local government offices.
5. Population: — average age of farmers; number of households headed by women; number of families and average size; number of children of pre-school age.	Census data; Statistics Unit.
6. Food Production and Availability: How the people get their food: — main crops grown (by season); livestock; home gardens; how food is stored/preserved; food supply eating patterns; beliefs and attitudes; child-feeding practices.	People in the community; local markets; local leaders; the agricultural centre; Young Farmers Clubs; local shops; health, community development and social workers.

Keeping records

All these topics are related to nutrition and health. Writing down the information, in other words, keeping records or reports can help you discover important facts about the community.

For example, collecting information on foods like what foods are available, how much and at what cost, is a good way to find out about community nutrition. You may see that certain crops are grown more at certain times of the year and less at others.

This type of information will help you understand some of the problems and needs of people in the community and help them plan suitable actions to overcome these problems.

An example of a record which could be kept is a calendar of food production and availability which shows the types of food crops and the seasons when they are grown. It also shows the times of the year when shortages of certain foods occur.

A seasonal calendar of food production and availability
This is a simple chart which shows the times of year when certain common foods are produced and, therefore, most available. Keeping such a record for each household will allow you to see what foods are in short supply. You will then be able to advise the family on what foods to grow and when to plant them.

At the top of the chart write the name of the family and in the section headed 'Foods', enter names of foods commonly grown in your district.

The next section shows the months of the year when the foods are grown. For each food, put an 'X' under the month when it is grown. The months which are blank show the times when a particular food is not grown. You can show the family how and when to plant certain crops so that they will be able to provide these foods for themselves when they cannot buy them. If they plant the crops so that the times of reaping do not exactly coincide, this will ensure a regular supply of food.

Foods	J	F	M	A	M	J	J	A	S	O	N	D
Staple Foods:												
Banana/Plantain	x	x	x	x	x	x	x	x	x	x	x	x
Breadfruit			x	x	x				x	x	x	
Maize	x	x	x							x	x	x
Yam	x	x	x	x	x	x	x	x	x	x	x	x
Potato, Irish	x	x	x	x							x	x
Potato, sweet	x	x	x	x	x	x	x	x	x	x	x	x
Legumes:												
Cow peas												
Black eye }	x	x	x	x	x	x	x	x	x	x	x	x
Broad beans												
Pigeon peas	x	x	x							x	x	x
Ground nuts						x	x	x	x			
Leafy Vegetables:												
Cabbage	x	x	x	x	x				x	x	x	x
Spinach	x	x	x	x	x	x	x	x	x	x	x	x

Foods	J	F	M	A	M	J	J	A	S	O	N	D
Other Vegetables:												
Pumpkin			x	x	x							
Tomato, Okra, Sweet pepper, }	x	x	x	x	x	x	x	x	x	x	x	x
Fruits in Season:												
Citrus	x	x	x						x	x	x	x
Guava			x	x	x				x	x	x	x
Mango	x	x	x	x	x	x	x				x	x
Paw paw			x	x	x	x	x					
Pineapple	x	x	x	x	x	x			x	x	x	x

Finding out what people eat and what else they do to keep fit

There are several ways of finding out what people eat and other things they do to keep fit. For getting ideas on their eating you can:

— Watch or observe them as you visit homes, shop or generally move around in the community.
— Follow them around for a day.
— Ask them to recall or say what they ate the day before or during the last 24 hours. This is called a **24 hour recall**.
— Ask or observe what they usually buy; what they get from the garden or other source; what's in the cupboard, safe or other storage area. When you do this, you make an **inventory**.
— Ask them to write down what they eat over several days,weeks or months. This is a **diet record**.
— Look at their grocery store cash register slip or grocery book.
— Even look at their peelings, empty cans, boxes or other food wrappers that they put in the garbage.
— Weigh the foods they eat before and after cooking and portions served. Find out how food is shared.

Finding out some of this information will take a lot of skill and time and may be awkward for you and people in the community.

However, there are ways to get around this problem, such as:

(a) Finding out the number of servings of foods from the six food groups that they eat at each meal or in a day, plus extras such as sugar, seasonings and alcoholic beverages.

How much families regard as a portion or serving of food may not be the same as you think. Notice the size of the dishes and utensils commonly used. You may have to weigh or measure a few portions as served to get an 'average size'.

(b) Finding out how often a food is eaten during a day or a week (**food frequency**) is another quick method. Ideas of usual amounts eaten can be assessed at the same time.

You can also ask about and observe activity and exercise patterns of people.

Here is a sample of a simple form which you can use for information on diet (eating) and activity pattern. We call this information a **diet/activity history**.

A DIET/ACTIVITY HISTORY FORM

Name ....

Address .... Age ....

Height ...... Weight ...... Occupation ....

Foods usually bought ....

Foods usually grown ....

Foods eaten or fed most days ....

Approx. amounts of food eaten ....

Where eaten (home, work, restaurant, school, other) ....

Foods disliked ....

Cooking, fuel, water facilities ....

Vitamins or other supplements taken ....

Exercise taken regularly (walking, jogging, skipping, dancing, etc.)

....

Times per week exercise done ....

For how long is exercise taken each time ....

Sports engaged in (give names) ....

About how many hours sleep daily ....

Last time visited doctor, health centre, diet counsellor

....

IDENTIFYING AND SOLVING PROBLEMS

The background information you have collected will help in identifying the most important food and nutrition problems as seen by the community, e.g. food shortages, malnutrition, obesity and anaemia and the factors involved. After collecting the information, you should meet with the people and discuss it. Meetings and discussions with individuals or groups are useful for helping people look closely at the reasons for problems. They need to understand why problems do or do not occur so that they will be able to choose the best actions to take to solve their problems. People in the community, other community workers and health staff at clinics/health centres/hospitals are examples of some of these people with whom you will discuss the problems.

The aim of these discussions is to learn as much as possible about the problems — how they are regarded by each group, the number of people who have these problems, the behaviour that causes the problems, possible reasons for this behaviour, other causes of the problems, what solutions are possible, what are the best solutions, how these solutions will fit into people's lives, the advantages and disadvantage of each solution and so on.

Suggesting causes for food and nutrition problems

There are many reasons why food and nutrition problems occur and it is important to try and identify the most important causes. Some of these may be:
— not enough food for everyone but especially for young children;
— too little money to buy food;
— no jobs;
— not enough education;
— bad roads and no transportation to take crops to the market;
— not enough clean, safe water;
— infections and diseases in children;
— poor families with too many children.

Often nutrition problems are caused also by bad practices such as:
— poor handling and storage of food,
— unsanitary disposal of rubbish and human waste.
— improper weaning practices.

You need to work with the community in finding out possible causes for the problems as well as possible reasons for the bad practices which cause problems.

Developing a plan of action

Since problems often have several causes, the community must decide on different actions to take in solving them. Deciding on which actions to take will depend on the kind of problem, its causes and the reasons behind the behaviours which cause it. A plan for taking action will involve:

— understanding and stating clearly what you want to achieve.
— deciding on the activities and materials you will need.
— identifying the people you will need.
— giving jobs or tasks to people.
— putting the whole plan into a time-frame which shows when the activities will start and end.

EVALUATION

Evaluation can mean three things: (1) Checking on, or monitoring how well a plan is being carried out, or how well the different activities which are part of the plan, are going; (2) Examining or measuring the final results of an activity; (3) Examining the costs involved in carrying out the plan or activity, how much time was involved and whether the money spent justified the results achieved.

Evaluation should be based on the views of everyone who was involved in planning and in carrying out the activities. You may carry out evaluation either verbally or in writing. However, you should write down the results carefully so that you will have a record of what happened. Your notes will also help you plan and carry out future programmes more effectively.

Evaluation must be done:

— from different points of view (e.g. the community worker; community members; other community workers; people from outside);
— clearly and frankly;
— completely, giving both strong and weak points.

Why evaluate?

If at the beginning of a plan or activity, we have a clear idea of what we want, evaluation will help us find out if we have succeeded. For example, if we wanted to see fewer children becoming malnourished, we need to know at the beginning what are the bad practices which help malnutrition to occur, also other causes. The plan of action to be followed will be aimed at changing these practices and correcting the other causes. Evaluating the results will show whether the bad practices which cause malnutrition are fewer and if there are more of the right behaviours which keep people healthy. Remember, it may take some time for the results of an activity to show, depending on the kind of health or nutrition problem which is being dealt with.

Evaluation is also important because:
— We can find out which actions will gain results and which will not.
— We can avoid repeating mistakes and help others to avoid the mistakes we have made.
— We can save time and money by not carrying on with unsuccessful activities.
— We can gain satisfaction by showing results.

Asking questions like:
— What things went well?
— Why did they go well?
— What new behaviours have people learned?
— How can they use these behaviours to solve other problems?
will help you and the community evaluate and learn from a plan or activity. If the results were not what you expected, you should try to find out why. Questions like these will help:
— Were there any problems in carrying out the activity?
— Did each person involved know what to do?
— Could each person do what he had to do?
— Did each person do what he had to do?
— How did he do it?
— Were the right kinds of activities chosen?

Answering these questions will help you and the community plan better activities and programmes for the future.

SUMMARY

Know your community   Find out what people do for a living; their backgrounds; interests; customs, etc., community organizations; services; population groups.

Assess the food and nutrition situation   Identify the chief food and nutrition problems and the factors which cause them. Consider possible sources of information on food and nutrition problems. Know how to keep records.

Know the different steps to follow in solving problems	Identify the chief problem. List causes of and possible solutions to the problem. Develop a plan of action and carry out activities which will help solve the problem. Evaluate the results.
Know how to develop and carry out a plan of action	State what you want to achieve Decide: What will be done Who will be involved What activities and methods will be used What will be needed When it will start and end
Be able to evaluate a plan or activity	Find out if people feel differently about the problem, understand more about the problem and have adopted the required change. Compare the results of an activity with what you wanted to achieve. Decide whether the methods used were the most appropriate. Identify the strong and weak points. Show how it could be improved the next time you do it. Write down the results.

2

Working with the community

Working with individuals in the community

Working with community groups

Working with other sectors

Summary

Child Development
Education
General

WHAT YOU SHOULD BE ABLE TO DO AFTER STUDYING THIS CHAPTER

This chapter will show you how to:
— Develop good relationships with people in the community.
— Help people in the community organize themselves in order to solve problems.
— Co-operate with other community workers in the community.

WORKING WITH INDIVIDUALS IN THE COMMUNITY

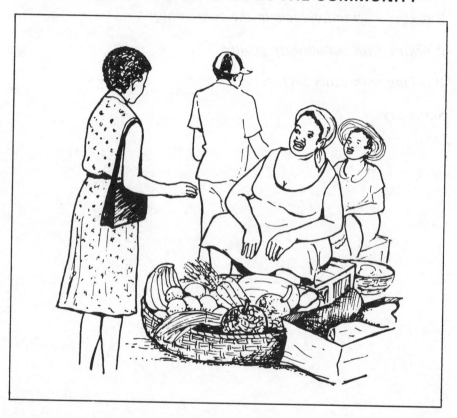

Some people do not belong to any special group in the community, but can be reached at places where they usually go to work, for example, washing by the riverside; at the shop or market or just along the street. This can be a useful way of exchanging information, finding out about coming events such as a meeting or talking about problems. As you get to know your community better, you will think of other ways of meeting people.

WORKING WITH COMMUNITY GROUPS

One of the ways in which a community worker can help people solve their problems is by helping them organize themselves into groups and work together to accomplish a common goal.

Benefits of working through groups:
— It encourages co-operation with other people and enables them to accomplish things which they would not be able to do alone.
— It provides contact with other people so that members can increase their knowledge and experience.
— It encourages participation and involvement in solving common problems.
— It develops the skills and talents of individual members.

Organizing community members into groups works best when there are problems which affect most people, for example, no piped water, not enough food, no health centre, no credit (loans) for farmers. Forming community groups helps community members agree on common problems and recognize that they can solve those problems by themselves, with outside help as needed.

The community worker should meet at first with individuals, then with larger and larger groups of people. This will help to identify the right leadership for building community awareness and responsibility for solving problems. This process of building leadership starts by asking such simple questions as 'Why do people get sick?', 'What can be done about it?' This is a slow process but it helps community members to begin to see that their problems can solved by them. It also helps the right kind of leadership to emerge.

Once leadership is created, the person takes responsibility for talking to more and more people about problems which everybody experiences. Once a group is formed it should start thinking about some sort of organization, with officers, a system of conducting meetings and plans for carrying out activities. The group should be quite clear as to why it came together in the first place. It must then develop and carry out plans to solve the community problems which brought it together.

Several groups may already be present in the community. They can help the community worker identify local problems. They can also be better organized to carry out tasks which are related to improving the food and nutrition situation. Members of these groups already have a history of working together and knowing their community and its problems. Community organizations like church groups, women's clubs, youth clubs, service clubs, schools and parent teachers' associations, farmers' groups and Health Committees are some examples. The community worker should try to get nutrition information to these groups at their regular meetings to get them interested and eager to help. The community worker should also identify the people who are most trusted and whose examples others will tend to follow. These are the people most likely to assume leadership in helping to make community members more aware of problems and consider what they can do to solve them. Let them guide you, then combine your ideas with theirs to reach effective solutions.

Keeping groups together

All groups come together for a special reason. Members of a group should agree on the reason why the group was formed and what is to be achieved. They should also feel closely involved in the activities which the group plans to carry out and that they have something to contribute. For groups to work well they need to develop clear plans of action.

How to develop a plan of action for a group:
— decide and write down what is to be accomplished;
— ask group members what are their interests and what resources they can contribute to the activity;
— make a list of all the things which need to be done (tasks);
— write down the tasks in the order in which they should be carried out (the priority), the length of time each will take and their relative importance;
— decide what is needed for the various taks (e.g. time, money, skills, etc.);
— divide the labour for carrying out tasks among group members, assigning jobs to people in line with their abilities and preferences;
— set deadlines (the dates by which tasks should be completed);
— evaluate the activities.

WORKING WITH OTHER SECTORS

On page 8, we saw that there are many reasons why food and nutrition problems exist.

Generally, these problems cannot be solved by any one agency, institution or sector working alone.

How different sectors help in solving food and nutrition problems

Health workers:
— monitoring nutritional status, for example, by growth charts;
— counselling chronically ill persons such as those with diabetes and hypertension;
— promoting good child and family feeding practices and wise use of family resources;
— promoting breastfeeding;
— preventing and treating illnesses and diseases, such as diarrhoea; malnutrition; obesity and anaemia;
— making contact with other agencies which could help families.

Agricultural extension workers:
— keeping checks on food production and availability;
— encouraging families to produce more food so as to increase incomes;
— promoting proper food production, marketing, storage, preparation and budgeting;
— promoting proper food distribution in the family;
— making contact with other agencies which could help families.

Community development workers:
— monitoring standards of living;
— helping families improve their homes and surroundings;
— promoting income-generating activities, especially for women;
— promoting good nutritional practices and use of family resources;
— developing community awareness of food and nutrition problems;
— building community organizations to solve problems.

School teachers:
— educating parents and school children on good nutritional practices and wise use of family resources;
— encouraging local food production through Young Farmers Clubs and school gardens;
— monitoring the health of school children;
— promoting good hygiene and sanitation;
— advising parents on the help which other agencies can provide.

Reasons for working with other sectors

Food and nutrition work in the community is often lonely and

discouraging. If community workers co-operate with colleagues who are running other programmes, they will be able to:
— combine resources;
— combine ideas;
— save on expenses;
— be a member of a group with common goals;
— share information about the community, and on plans and projects;
— plan together to avoid conflict;
— discuss problems and opportunities with others doing similar jobs;

A co-ordinate group of community workers can be far more effective than workers on their own. Workers can share transportation on field visits, record information in a way that others can use, and work towards common goals decided upon between the local community and themselves.

It is not always easy to achieve good communication and close co-operation with other field workers. Some reasons may be:
— age and sex differences;
— the fear that co-operation may result in shared, or even no credit for work done;
— unwillingness to co-operate at headquarters level;
— time and transport problems.

One way of solving these problems is to meet regularly with other community workers in the course of work, or socially. This will help to keep everyone informed about everyone else's programmes and projects. Community workers should also try to work together on individual projects. For example, a nutrition worker can gather information about vaccinations for the health worker as she visits homes. Or a women's club organized by different community workers can include health education, adult literacy and nutrition training in its programme

You should make a deliberate effort to work with other organizations, combining programmes wherever possible. This is called 'co-ordination'. The following situations show what happens when co-ordination is lacking.
— A field worker successfully persuades all the mothers in a village to give their children a nutritious diet. The children continue to suffer from diarrhoea. Why? Because the local water supply remains polluted.
— A field worker is asked to start a poultry project with the help of the school nutrition club. The children do not seem to have enough time to work on the project. Why? Because the headmaster had already introduced a school food production project in which the children have to spend a lot of their time.

Both examples show that the actions were carried out in isolation. The group involved did not combine or integrate their approaches to the problem. This caused the people concerned to become frustrated and confused.

When this happens people may not wish to try again. They may well ignore future attempts to help them, even if the future attempts are better planned, integrated and more likely to succeed.

Here are some examples of situations which show how important it is for people to work together:

— A nutrition officer tries to persuade people to build fish ponds to improve their diet. Later that day a health worker advises the same people to drain pools of water so that mosquitoes cannot breed. The people are confused, do not know which advice to follow and do nothing.

— A community development worker starts a campaign to persuade mothers to burn or bury all their household waste to improve hygiene. At the same time, the agricultural extension officer advises farmers to keep their household waste to make compost for their fields.

— A community development worker organizes a meeting to talk about plans for a pre-school, day care centre. Very few mothers attend the meeting. The worker finds out later that an important government official visited the village on the same day to talk about the coming election.

Problems like these can arise when there is no communication and co-operation between field workers.

The examples show that community groups which work well together can achieve more than each group working on its own.

There are several advantages in working closely with other community workers.

Developing communication and co-operation involves:

— finding opportunities for working together, either on community development committees or on individual projects;

— being aware of individual differences in personality and job responsibilities;

— having a common language;

— sharing responsibilities;

— sharing rewards;

— achieving something with others rather than by yourself.

— collecting information and recording it so that others can use it and using information others have collected;

— sharing information on plans and projects so that they do not clash.

What can you do as a member of an informal group of community workers?

— Find opportunities for working together, either on community development committees or on individual projects;
— Be aware of individual differences in personality and job responsibilities;
— Be aware that people's training, knowledge and responsibilities are different from yours, and that others know more about some aspects of the community than you do. Show them you accept this, want to learn and are willing to take advice. Do not pretend that you know things that you do not.
— 'Build bridges' among the group. For example, use the same words and terms.
— Co-operate together on small things first until you have had some practice. You may want to share a meal to which each person brings some food or drink. Then move into the area of community work, undertaking simple, then more complex activities. Remember you will all have your individual responsibilities.
— Limit the group at first to a practical size. Even two workers acting together is better than one acting alone.
— Equally share responsibilities, duties and rewards.
— Try to co-operate on things that will give everyone an equal share of rewards or results as individuals.
— If someone refuses to join you, do not pressure him but leave the offer open.
— Always act professionally. Concentrate on achieving something with the community rather than on who or what you are.

Building communication and co-operation with other sectors, agencies and institutions working in the community is a great asset.

When people work together, they gain the confidence of the local community. They save scarce resources by combining their efforts. They get support and encouragement from their colleagues and share problems with them. This makes community work less of a lonely task.

SUMMARY

Develop good relationships with people in the community	Seek out and work with influential persons and groups in the community. Help to build community awareness and responsibility for solving problems.

Work with individuals in the community	Reach people in places of work; social meetings.
Help people organize themselves into groups	Identify local leadership. Work with groups in identifying common problems and their solutions. Help groups develop work plans.
Identify roles of different sectors in improving the food and nutrition situation in the community	Identify the roles of health, agricultural extension and community development workers, also school teachers, which can help to improve the food and nutrition situation. Co-operate with them in playing these roles better.
Practise good team work. Develop ways of communicating and co-operating with community workers	Share information on plans and projects. Combine resources, ideas and expenses. Join an informal group of community workers which meet regularly. Share responsibilities and duties within the group.

3
Planning food and nutrition education programmes

Applying communication to food and nutrition education

Planning nutrition education programmes

Summary

**Food and Nutrition
Education
Child development
General**

WHAT YOU SHOULD BE ABLE TO DO AFTER STUDYING THIS CHAPTER

This chapter will show you how to:
— Plan nutrition education programmes.
— Develop, pre-test and communicate messages.
— Choose the right methods for communicating messages.

APPLYING COMMUNICATION TO FOOD AND NUTRITION EDUCATION

Food and Nutrition Education is a process by which people gain the knowledge, attitudes, confidence and skills necessary for developing good dietary practices.

Communication is sharing ideas, information, attitudes, values or instructions with individuals or with groups to help people choose the behaviours and make the changes which are best for them. It involves both giving and receiving information. The community worker who communicates well must not only give information to the community but also listen carefully to what the community is saying.

Communication alone cannot solve problems but it will help to involve people actively in making the changes which will improve their lives.

It can be applied to any field or activity which is aimed at change, for example, to food and nutrition education, which aims to help people change wrong behaviours and adopt those behaviours which lead to better health.

PLANNING NUTRITION EDUCATION PROGRAMMES

The steps to be followed in planning and carrying out nutrition education programmes are the same ones to be followed in solving problems.

However, there are some other factors to be considered in planning and carrying out nutrition education programmes. These are the specific groups of people you may want to reach, the kind of information you want to give them and the ways in which the information may be given.

Identifying people to be reached
Information collected about the community, its problems and their

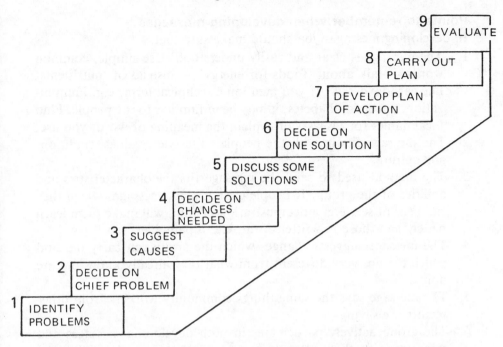

causes will allow you to identify and describe the people who are most affected by food and nutrition problems and who you will want to reach. Discussing these problems with them will help you to find out both what they want and need in order to improve their lives. Understanding how the problems affect them will help you suggest the kind of help they may need. One kind of help could be food and nutrition education.

Community workers from other sectors should also be contacted to learn of their experiences in dealing with similar problems and groups of people.

Developing messages
From the information gathered you will be able to develop a series of 'messages' — the kind of information which will help people solve their food and nutrition problems.

Some examples of messages which relate to common food and nutrition problems in the community may be:
— grow and eat more leafy vegetables;
— breastfeed babies for at least four months;
— give oral rehydration salts (ORS) as soon as diarrhoea appears;
— give other foods as well as breastmilk to children from four months;
— grow and eat more cowpeas, beans and ground nuts
— keep a backyard garden.

Points to remember when developing messages

In developing messages you should make sure that:

1. The message is clear and easily understood. Use simple, common words — talk about 'foods for energy' — instead of 'nutritients' like carbohydrates. If you mention a technical term, e.g. immunization, anaemia, diabetes, it may be unfamiliar to the people. Find local names for diseases or explain the meaning of words you use.

2. The message fits in with the people's lifestyles, values, traditions and culture.

3. The method used to send the message fits the characteristics and abilities of the group. If people cannot read, messages which they can hear or see, e.g. a demonstration or film, will make them learn better than those in written form, e.g. a pamphlet.

4. The message suggests changes which the group can carry out and which are not very different from what they already know and are doing.

5. The message says the same things community workers from other sectors are saying.

6. The group actively participates in both developing messages and responding to them. People must be involved in describing the problem as seen by them, and the message must be developed from this information.

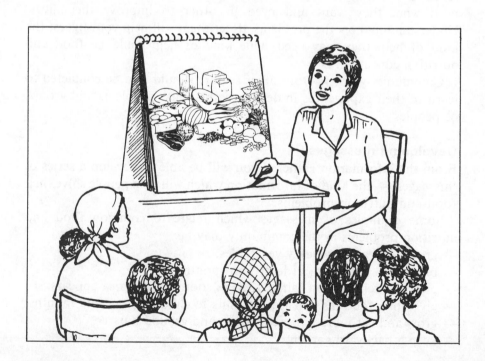

Pre-testing messages

People should also be asked questions to find out if they understand a message, like the way it is put and can carry out the changes it suggests. This is called pre-testing. Pre-testing messages with a small number of people helps to make sure that a message is well suited to the group for which it is intended. You can also pre-test methods and materials to find out if they work in the way they were planned. After asking questions and getting answers, you will need to make changes to the message, method or materials, according to the suggestions you have received.

Communicating messages

Messages may be sent by:
— the spoken word, e.g. a conversation, discussion or public meeting;
— the written word, e.g. books, letters, reports, newspapers, magazines;
— visuals, e.g. diagrams, pictures, drawings, photographs, slides;
— action, e.g. drama, demonstration, field days.

These may be used either separately or together. For example, the spoken word can be combined with movement, as in television, films or plays; action can be combined with visuals, as in an exhibition. In general, communication is always more successful if we use a mixture of methods, e.g. talking while we do a demonstration; showing posters during a talk.

Before choosing a method of communicating messages you should make sure that it suits the people, their circumstances and the problem to be solved.

One or more of these methods can be used during your day-to-day work in the community, e.g. in conversations — during home visits and when meeting people informally; in formal meetings; in discussions and in demonstrations. Some techniques for good communication in these situations will be discussed in the next chapter.

A plan of action for communicating messages also needs to be developed as part of the whole nutrition education programme. It will involve:
— the number of times each message needs to be repeated over a period;
— the ways in which messages will be sent, e.g. discussions, demonstrations, field days, exhibitions, public meetings;
— the resources needed to communicate the messages, e.g. transport, demonstration materials, audio-visual aids, mass media, other people;
— the times when each message will be communicated and how long it

will take;
— the effect of the message on the target group.

SUMMARY

Know the steps in planning food and nutrition education programmes

Collect information about the community. Identify food and nutrition problems. Decide on the chief problem. Suggest causes for the problem and possible solutions. Decide on one solution. Develop a plan of action. Identify the people to be reached. Develop and pre-test messages. Choose the right methods for communicating messages. Evaluate the results.

Identify people to be reached

Identify people in the community who are experiencing food and nutrition problems. Learn all about these people. Find out what they want and need to know and do. Find out what they already know, and what they are already doing. Use this information to develop messages.

Learn to communicate well

Be clear and specific about what you plan to do in the community. Listen to what people have to say and change messages accordingly. Understand the people you want to reach. Choose the right methods in dealing with different groups of people. Make sure people understand what you are telling them. Make sure that people can do what you want them to do. Ask people to tell you how they feel about what you are telling them.

Know how to develop and pre-test messages

Messages developed should: Be clear and understandable. Relate to community problems. Fit in with community lifestyles. Suggest benefits to be gained by

	the intended change. Be pre-tested on a section of the intended group to get their reactions, then changed accordingly.
Be able to choose the best methods for communicating messages	Messages may be communicated verbally, in writing, through drawings or by actions. A mixture of methods is better than one method used alone.

4

Some techniques of good communication

Education
Child Development
General

WHAT YOU SHOULD BE ABLE TO DO AFTER STUDYING THIS CHAPTER

This chapter will show you how to:
— Communicate clearly during:
- Informal conversations
- Home visits
- Talks
- Informal meetings and discussions
- Demonstrations
— Evaluate your performance.

COMMUNICATING CLEARLY

During the course of your job as a community worker, you may encounter a number of situations during which food and nutrition ideas, information and advice will be communicated. Having good communication skills and practising good communication techniques will help you to handle these situations more effectively.

Having communication skills means how well a person (the sender) can listen, think, draw, speak, write or act in any other way in the communication process. It also means how well the audience can listen, read, and use all relevant senses in getting messages. The aim of good communication is to make sure that individuals or groups can hear, see and understand clearly the message that is being shared with them.

The communication process

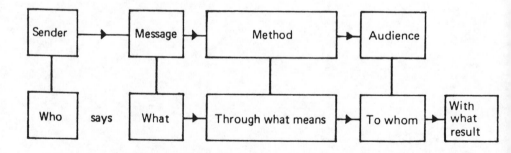

Ideas for communicating clearly
1. Know your audience — the people with whom you will be communicating. Build a good relationship with them.
2. Be sure that your messages suit the audience — use words and ideas

that the people can understand well. Talk about things which are familiar to them.

3. Choose the right methods for communicating messages.
4. Listen to your audience. Remember, communication is both giving and receiving. How the audience responds and reacts is an important part of the communication process. It tells us whether or not the messages are understood and how the people feel about what they heard or saw.
5. Be sure that messages are communicated in a place convenient for the intended audience, under the best possible conditions and at the right time, e.g. when having a discussion make sure the room is quiet and not crowded. If you plan to meet with women, find out when they go out to work and when they are at home.

Some of the situations you will encounter in which good communication skills and techniques will be helpful are:

INFORMAL CONVERSATIONS

Informal conversations can take place on the street, in places where people meet and in their homes during home visits. In such situations, you may talk casually or informally about several different subjects. Or you may want to get information about a particular subject and will have a plan in mind, even though the meeting is still informal. It is important to be prepared.

Holding informal conversations is a good way of getting the views of a number of people on a particular subject. You will need to prepare, either a rough outline of the discussion you plan to have, or a number of questions which you want to ask.

Good communication is extremely important. You need to establish an atmosphere of friendliness and ease with the person with whom you are talking. This way you are most likely to get the person to co-operate in answering questions.

Points to remember
— Be friendly and courteous.
— Explain why you want to talk to that person.
— Show interest in whatever is said without giving your opinion.
— Repeat questions in a different way to try to make them clearer if the person does not understand.
— Listen well and try to hear 'what is not being said' as well as the spoken words.
— Find time for a few minutes of friendly chat before leaving.
— When you go home, write down the chief points of the conversation.

HOME VISITS

One of the tasks of a community worker is to visit people in their homes. During these visits, you will talk informally to members of the family to share ideas and information with them. This is one of the best ways of getting to know about people, and letting the family members get to know you.

There are many advantages in making a home visit. You can watch the family do things they have learned at the Health Centre, Young Farmers Club, school or on an agricultural field day. You can learn from what they do or say. You can teach them new things. You may go because they have asked for help or because someone told you they needed help.

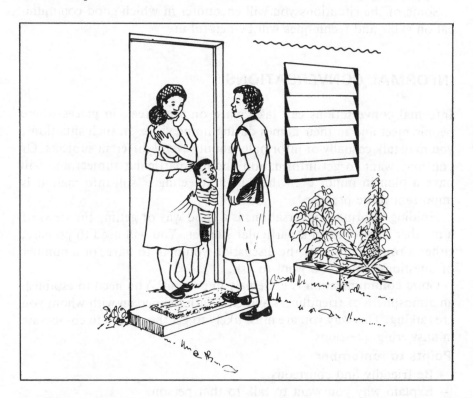

Your first visit will be to find out more about the family and let them get to know you.

How to make your home visit useful
— Plan for it. Have a reason for making the visit. Think about all the methods you can use which will help to make the visit interesting.
— Be friendly and sympathetic. Always find something to praise. Start

the conversation by asking about the family. Remember people's names. Be a good listener and close observer. Try to make them trust you and don't do anything that will make them lose faith in you.

> **Don't tell anyone what the family tells you in confidence.**

— Be sure you and the family understand each other and that you all understand and agree on any plans you make for the future. After you have left the house, write down the things you want to remember. Do not forget to do the things you promised to do during your visit. Here is a sample of a form which can be used for recording home visits:

HOME VISIT RECORD

Name: ....

Address: ....

Family members: ....

Ages: ....

1. The Visit:
   (a) What I planned to do: ....
   (b) What I did: ....
   (c) What the family agreed to do: ....
   (d) What I promised to do for follow-up: ....

2. The situation — special problems if any ....
   ....

3. Materials or information promised ....

4. Proposed date of next visit: ....

                                    Date: ....

TALKS

Talks are usually given to get across a particular idea or practice.

A talk should be given at a time when the audience most needs that specific information. The information must be practical, based on facts and suitable for the intended audience.

Presenting ideas clearly during a talk depends very much on how the information has been organized. After you have collected the information, spend some time putting it in proper order. Then practise giving the talk, either in front of the mirror, on friends or members of your family.

Points to remember when giving a talk
— Dress appropriately for the occasion.
— Tell the audience what you plan to say and do.
— Make sure that people are comfortable and at ease. Relax the group by telling stories or jokes, but be careful with this technique as not many people have the skill to do it well.
— Be sure that everyone can see and hear properly.
— Talk 'to' not 'at' people. This does not mean talking down to them — but respecting them as persons in their own right.
— Encourage people to take part. Either stop from time to time and ask for comments or plan a question-and-answer session at the end of your talk.
— Be confident. Don't apologise for your shortcomings. Don't worry about being nervous. Try to speak out naturally in a loud, clear voice and **be yourself**.
— During the talk **observe your audience**. Check to see whether people are getting bored or losing interest. If they are, try to make your talk a little livelier or encourage the audience to take part at that point.
— Never memorize a speech. Plan a 'content outline' on small cards or sheets of paper. Use these instead of long sheets of paper to refer to during the talk.
— If possible, use visual aids, like charts, posters or pictures, to add interest to your talk. A demonstration is useful if you are teaching the group how to do something.
— If possible have something to give away — leaflets, samples, etc. after your talk.
— Time yourself. Be as brief as possible while making important points. **Stop** while the audience's interest is high.
— Avoid annoying gestures and mannerisms which could be distracting.
— Be lively and appear interested in your subject.

FORMAL MEETINGS AND DISCUSSIONS

In formal meetings and discussions, there is an exchange of ideas on one topic and more than one person takes part. A discussion is different from a conversation in that it usually has a special focus. Someone should lead or be in charge and remarks should be addressed to that person.

How to lead a discussion
— Choose the right atmosphere so that everyone can see, hear and think clearly.
— Open the discussion in such a way that participants are at ease and ready to take part. Give a brief explanation of the topic. This might include:
  (a) why the subject is being discussed at that time;
  (b) importance of subject being discussed.
— Encourage participants to put forward their ideas so that as many ideas as possible can be considered.
— Invite participants to ask questions.
— If the discussion slows down, throw out questions to start participants thinking again, but be sure to avoid questions with a simple 'yes' or 'no' answer.
— If you are playing a leadership role, do not try to answer questions or challenges from the participants. Listen to the discussion without putting forward your own views.
— From time to time, it is useful to sum up what has been covered by the discussion up to that point. But be very careful not to add any new ideas of your own.
— Discourage interruptions.
— Keep the discussion on the subject.
— Keep a watch on the time so that the discussion can be completed promptly.
— Give each one a fair chance to make his/her point.

DEMONSTRATIONS

A demonstration shows people new skills and is a lively way of combining practical examples with facts. People can see, hear, talk about and take part in a demonstration. This helps them learn better than if they just sat and listened to a talk.

Here is what a good demonstration should do:
— Teach skills which people want to learn.
— Take place at the right time, e.g. planting food at the right season, preserving fruits when they are reaped, learning about weaning when the child is at the right age, etc.

— Use the things that are familiar to the people and which they can afford and can practise, e.g. in a cooking demonstration, use the kinds of pots and cooking fuel that the women have in their kitchens.

How to carry out a good demonstration
— Plan the demonstration.
— Introduce yourself and explain the ideas and skills which you will be demonstrating. Use pictures, posters or photographs to give the group a clear idea of what to expect.
— Find out what the people expect to get and modify your plan accordingly.
— Make the demonstration look simple enough for others to do it. Do each step slowly, one at a time. Make sure everyone can see.
— Talk to your audience while you are doing the demonstration.
— Encourage questions.
— Look at the audience while you work.
— Speak loudly and clearly and use simple language.
— Ask questions to test people's understanding. Repeat the steps if people do not understand them.
— If possible, ask one person to repeat the demonstration and ask the group to comment as the person works. Go over the important points and give suggestions for improvement.
— Ask questions to make sure people understand.
— Give everyone a chance to practise.
— Tell people where they can get supplies and equipment, handouts, recipes or other materials.
— Be clear about what you will do next or what you expect them to do next.
— If this is one of a set of demonstrations, tell them when the next one will be. At the beginning of the next session ask one of the group to repeat the preceding demonstration. This will test how much they remembered.

HOW TO EVALUATE YOUR PERFORMANCE

Evaluation should be done both during and after all your everyday activities as a community worker. The following questions will help you think about your performance and how it could be improved:
During the activity:
— Did you talk to people and listen to them?
— Did you make an effort to establish good relationships and communicate clearly?

— Did you help people see the reasons for this activity and other factors?
— Did you ask people to give their own ideas for solving the problems?
— Did you help them choose the actions best suited to their circumstances?

At the end of the activity:

— Did people learn new knowledge, ideas and skills as well as was planned?
— Can the people practise the skills they were taught?
— Are there changes in people's behaviour?
— Are there signs that the problem is being solved?

Some time after the activity:

— Are the people able to put their new skills to use?
— Are there changes in people's behaviour?
— Has the problem been solved?
— Could they have done anything differently or better?
— What could you have done differently to help people acquire new skills/make changes/solve problems?
— What could have been done in the same way?

SUMMARY

Communicate clearly	Know your audience. Be sure that your messages suit the audience. Choose the right methods for communicating messages. Listen to your audience.
Know how to meet people informally	Greet people politely and talk to them in a way they understand and appreciate. Explain why you want to talk. Show interest in whatever is said.
Know how to make home visits	Develop a plan. Keep in confidence what people tell you. Do for people what you promised you would do. Keep appointments or cancel them in good time. Keep a home visit record.
Know how to conduct formal meetings and discussions	Make sure people are relaxed and ready to participate. Encourage people to put their ideas forward. Keep the discussion on the subject. Summarize the discussion.

Know how to plan and deliver a talk	Organize your information. Practise giving your talk, on family or friends. Tell the audience what you plan to say and do. Encourage people to take part. Observe people's reactions.
Know how to carry out demonstrations	Make a simple plan and follow it. Involve the audience in the demonstration. Use the things people usually have and can afford. Make sure people have understood the demonstration.
Know how to evaluate your own performance	Did you encourage people's participation in identifying and solving problems? Did the people learn new skills/make changes/solve problems? What could be done differently, better or in the same way?

5

Food and good health

What is food?

Using food groups as a guide to good nutrition

Food groups for the tropics

Meal planning with food groups
— The balanced diet principle

Ideas and suggestions for learning about
food and good health

Health
Food and Nutrition
Agriculture

WHAT YOU SHOULD BE ABLE TO DO
AFTER STUDYING THIS CHAPTER

After reading this chapter, taking part in discussions and doing the exercises and activities, you should be able to:
— Advise people on how food nourishes the body.
— Divide food into six common groups.
— Help people to understand the principle of a balanced diet.
— Help families plan meals according to the principle of a balanced diet.

WHAT IS FOOD?

What we eat and drink to help keep us alive and well, to help us grow, develop, work and play is called food. All living things need food. Food satisfies hunger and nourishes the body. Food gives us a feeling of comfort and satisfaction. Eating certain foods establishes our identity. For some of us this means eating the traditional foods of our parents and grandparents. For others it is buying expensive or prestigious food to show that we are better off economically. Food is also used to show friendship and love.

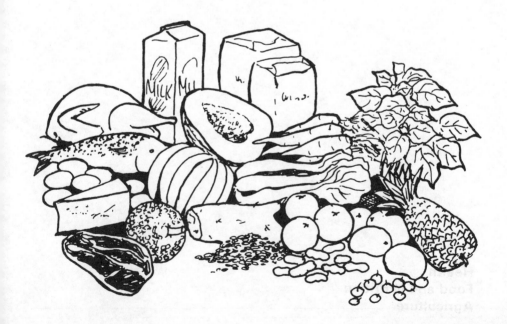

What we eat and how we eat makes up our food habits. Most of our food habits are learned in the home from our families. As we grow up our experiences help us to change some of these habits. Travel, new experiences and learning about nutrition can help us change food habits.

How food keeps us healthy

Every time we move we use energy. Even when we move slowly or appear to be resting, the mere act of living is using up energy. The heart keeps on beating; the lungs keep working; the blood keeps circulating throughout the body.

Food is needed to provide energy for work and warmth for the body. It is needed to build, maintain and repair the body. It is also required for control of body processes and for protection against diseases and infections. By performing these functions food helps us to keep healthy, warm, well-nourished and alive.

What food does for our bodies

Foods contain chemical substances called 'nutrients'. Nutrients are found in varying amounts and combinations in different foods.

This book is going to discuss the twelve most important nutrients. These are:

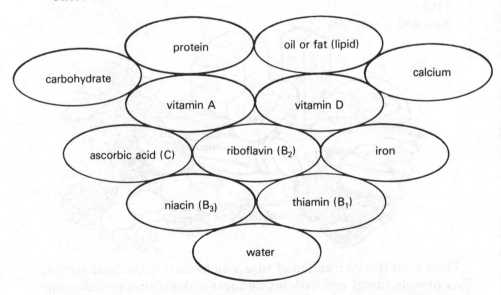

Enough food containing the twelve nutrients should be eaten every day. It's likely that you'll get enough of the other nutrients your body needs by doing this. No one food supplies all the nutrients the body needs. No one nutrient is most important. Each nutrient has certain jobs that it does in the body. The nutrients work together to keep us healthy.

Besides nutrients, foods contain fibre or roughage. Fibre is very important in the diet. It makes the bowels work properly and provides bulk to make us feel full. It's especially useful to people trying to lose weight, and to diabetics. Fresh fruits and vegetables, peas and beans, wholewheat flour and unrefined maize or sorghum flour give us fibre.

USING FOOD GROUPS AS A GUIDE TO GOOD NUTRITION

Good health starts with eating properly. Eating properly means eating enough of the right kinds of food.

There are guides to help us choose the right foods and eat healthy meals. The guide we use fits in very well with our way of preparing meals. This guide breaks the foods we usually eat into six big groups. These are:

1. Staples such as cereals, roots and tubers
2. Legumes (beans) and nuts
3. Dark green leafy and/or yellow vegetables
4. Food from animals
5. Fruits
6. Fats and substitutes

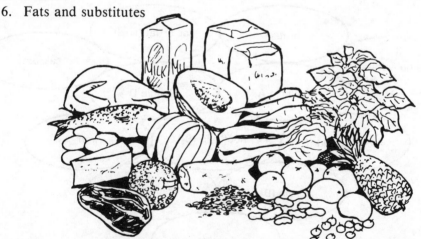

There is no special mention of sugars and sweets in the food groups. They provide energy and dark brown sugar and molasses provide some iron.

There are many foods in each group. The foods in each group are alike in some way. The following table shows common foods from which we get a good amount of some nutrients:

A QUICK GUIDE TO SOURCES OF NUTRIENTS*

This is a rough guide to the nutrient content of foods. However, all foods are mixtures of nutrients and only foods providing significant amount of a nutrient are listed.

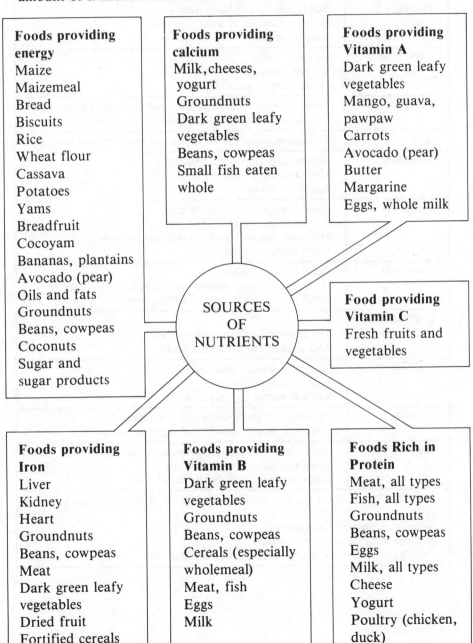

Foods providing energy
Maize
Maizemeal
Bread
Biscuits
Rice
Wheat flour
Cassava
Potatoes
Yams
Breadfruit
Cocoyam
Bananas, plantains
Avocado (pear)
Oils and fats
Groundnuts
Beans, cowpeas
Coconuts
Sugar and sugar products

Foods providing calcium
Milk, cheeses, yogurt
Groundnuts
Dark green leafy vegetables
Beans, cowpeas
Small fish eaten whole

Foods providing Vitamin A
Dark green leafy vegetables
Mango, guava, pawpaw
Carrots
Avocado (pear)
Butter
Margarine
Eggs, whole milk

SOURCES OF NUTRIENTS

Food providing Vitamin C
Fresh fruits and vegetables

Foods providing Iron
Liver
Kidney
Heart
Groundnuts
Beans, cowpeas
Meat
Dark green leafy vegetables
Dried fruit
Fortified cereals

Foods providing Vitamin B
Dark green leafy vegetables
Groundnuts
Beans, cowpeas
Cereals (especially wholemeal)
Meat, fish
Eggs
Milk

Foods Rich in Protein
Meat, all types
Fish, all types
Groundnuts
Beans, cowpeas
Eggs
Milk, all types
Cheese
Yogurt
Poultry (chicken, duck)

FUNCTIONS OF SOME NUTRIENTS

NUTRIENT	WHAT IT DOES
Fat	Supplies energy Carries fat-soluble vitamins A, D, E and K
Protein	Builds and repairs body tissues Builds antibodies to fight infection Supplies energy
Carbohydrate	Supplies energy Supplies fibre Helps body to use fats
Calcium	Helps to build bones and teeth and keep them strong Promotes healthy nerves and normal blood clotting
Iron	Transports oxygen in the body and helps prevent anaemia
Vitamin C	Maintains healthy teeth and gums Maintains strong blood vessel walls Assists in absorption of iron
Vitamin A	Helps bone and teeth to develop Promotes good night vision Maintains the health of the skin and membranes Helps fight infection
Vitamin D	Helps bones to grow strong Helps body to use calcium and phosphorus to make bones grow, repair them and form teeth
B VITAMINS: **Thiamin**	Releases energy from carbohydrate Aids normal growth and appetite
Riboflavin	Maintains healthy skin and eyes Maintains healthy nerves Releases energy to body cells
Niacin	Promotes normal growth and development Maintains healthy nerves and digestive system
Water	Carries nutrients to and wastes from the body cells Helps regulate body temperature Helps digestion and absorption of food

NOTE: Fibre is not a nutrient but it is very important for good health. It:
— helps to prevent constipation;
— helps some people to lose weight;
— helps to reduce the risk of heart disease and diabetes.

FOOD GROUPS IN THE TROPICS

We can choose the foods we like from the different groups. This guide tells us how to choose from each group.

1. Staples

These include the cereals and the starchy fruits, roots and tubers. These are very important in the tropical diets. They are prepared in many ways as the staple or main part of the meal.

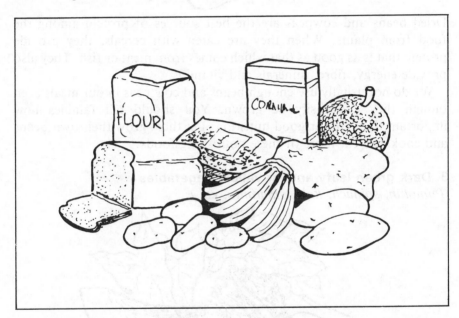

(a) *Cereal grains such as rice, maize, sorghum, millet, wheat, barley.*
    They give energy, protein, some B vitamins and some minerals. When cereals are processed to produce a fine product (like white flour) some of the food value is lost. This is because some of the nourishment is found in the coarse layers of the grain. Sometimes some of the nourishment lost is put back. The process of putting back nourishment is called enrichment. Some cereals (like whole wheat flour) have not had as much of the nourishment removed. They also have more fibre than highly refined cereals.

(b) *Starchy fruits, roots and tubers, such as plantain, breadfruit, yam, sweet potato, cassava, Irish potato, cocoyam.*
    Starchy fruits, roots and tubers have a lot of energy, but not much protein. Because of this, we should eat them whenever possible with foods which provide protein, such as food from animals, for example meat and fish.

2. Legumes and nuts

(Pigeon peas, cowpeas, beans, dahl, groundnuts, soya beans)

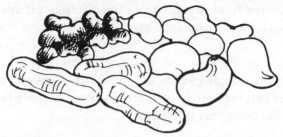

Dried beans and cowpeas are the best sources of protein among the food from plants. When they are eaten with cereals, they provide protein that is as good as that which comes from meat or fish. They also provide energy, fibre, minerals and vitamins.

We do not usually use enough beans and cow peas in our meals even though they can easily be grown. You should tell families how important they are for good nutrition. Let them grow their own beans and cook and eat more of these nourishing foods.

3. Dark green leafy and/or yellow vegetables

(Pumpkin, spinach, kale, amarantu, etc.)

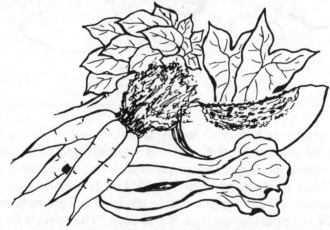

These vegetables are important because they contain a substance which can be changed in the body to vitamin A. The dark green leafy vegetables also contain iron. It is very important to eat plants which contain iron. When there is too little iron in the diet, a disease called anaemia (see page 143) occurs.

Dark green leafy vegetables also contain vitamin C, some minerals and protein. Each member of the family, even the youngest, should eat dark green or yellow vegetables each day.

Children should have as many of these vegetables as possible. Leafy vegetables also give the body fibre.

Other vegetables, such as squash, cucumbers and eggplants contain very little food value. They add bulk and are useful in the diets of those who need to control energy intake, such as obese people and diabetics.

4. Food from animals
(Eggs, fish, chicken, milk, cheese and meats)

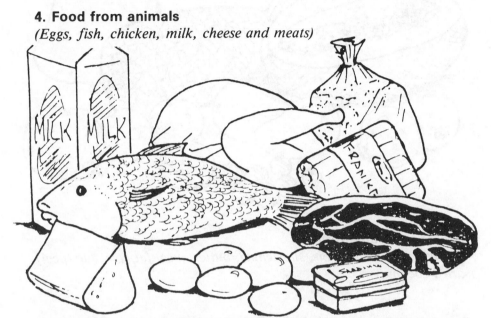

These foods are important for their good quality protein, minerals and vitamins. Milk and cheese also provide vitamin A and the B vitamin, riboflavin which is hardly found in other foods. Meats, especially heart, kidney and liver are important sources of iron. Most people enjoy eating meat and other foods from this group. Because they are expensive, people think they are more important than other foods. This is not true. You can have a good, well-balanced diet with only small amounts of food from animals.

5. Fruits
(Pawpaw, mango, guava, pineapple, orange, grapefruit, etc.)
Most fruits are a rich source of vitamin C, especially when eaten fresh. Vitamin C is important to help the body use the iron from other foods. Fruits or juices containing vitamin C, such as orange juice, should be taken with meals containing iron-rich foods. Some of these iron-rich foods are dark green leafy vegetables, peas, beans and meats.

Bright, yellow fleshy fruits like mango and ripe pawpaw also contain good amounts of carotene, a substance the body changes into vitamin A.

Fibre is also found in fresh fruits.

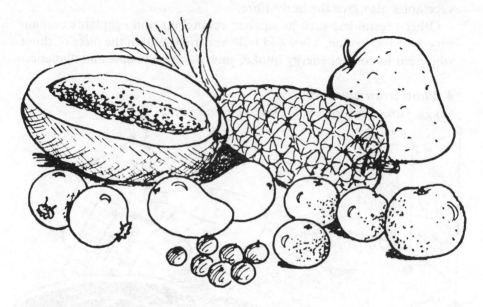

6. Fats and substitutes

(Cooking oils, margarine, shortening, butter, meat fat, avocado (pear), dried coconut)

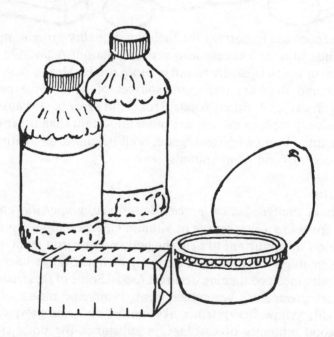

These foods are very good sources of energy. Butter and fortified margarine contain vitamin A. Most foods contain fat, although it is not always easily seen, for example the butterfat in regular milk, the fat in meats and some fish.

Fats are good to add to the foods given to the very young child when he is being weaned gradually from the breast to solid foods. Fats make foods taste good but we need to eat only a small amount. Vegetable oils are better than animal fats, which in large amounts can cause disease.

Other foods

Sugar and sweets

Sugars and sweets can also cause people to become overweight or get bad teeth. If children develop a taste for very sweet foods, they may get into the habit of eating foods that will cause them to become overweight adults. They may also not eat enough of more nutritious foods. Fresh fruits and sugar cane, which are naturally sweet, are better snacks than sweets.

MEAL PLANNING WITH FOOD GROUPS — THE PRINCIPLE OF BALANCED DIET

The principle of a balanced diet is a way to plan meals by combining foods from different groups, it helps people who prepare meals to give their families good nutrition. This principle can help families to make their usual meals more nutritious. The principle of a balanced diet teaches us that the foods we eat at each meal should come from the different food groups.

A balanced meal starts with a staple. This staple is served with foods from one or more of the other groups. Most family meals already contain foods from more than one group. A good balanced meal can be a one-pot meal of foods from at least three of the food groups, e.g. soup, or it can be a meal which contains separate dishes made from at least three of the food groups, e.g. rice + chicken + pumpkin.

The beverage which the family drinks with a meal can become part of a balanced diet if it is chosen from one of the food groups, for example a fruit or vegetable juice like carrot juice or soursop drink.

Meals from 4-6 food groups

The most nourishing meals will include foods from all six food groups or from the four chief food groups. For example, a meal of rice and peas, chicken and pumpkin is very nutritious. It includes:

Staple	+	Legumes and nuts	+	Dark green leafy/ yellow vegetables	+	Food from animals
Rice				Pumpkin		Chicken

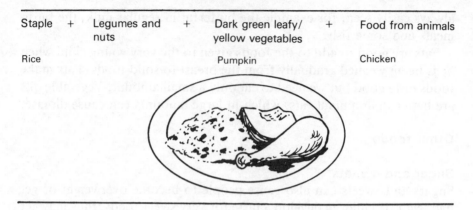

Some fat will be used in preparing the meal, e.g. oil for frying, and if fruit like pineapple or a tangerine is eaten with the meal, foods from all six groups would be included in the meal.

Meals from 3-4 food groups

A nourishing meal may also contain foods from three of the chief groups. This can be a little cheaper to make.

Examples of such meals are:

Staple	+	Dark green leafy yellow vegetables	+	Food from animals
Potato or yam		Spinach		Fish

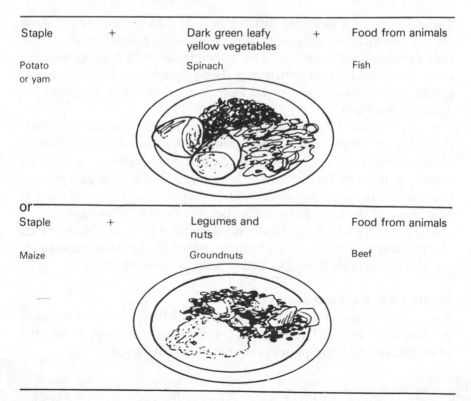

or

Staple	+	Legumes and nuts		Food from animals
Maize		Groundnuts		Beef

or

Staple	+	Legumes and nuts	+	Dark green leafy/ yellow vegetables
Cassava porridge		Cowpeas		Pumpkin

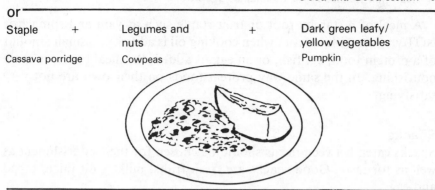

Usually cooking oil or margarine are used while preparing these meals. By adding fat you will use foods from four groups to make these meals.

Meals from 2-3 food groups

The cheapest meals may be made with foods from only two of the chief groups. It is important to choose such meals very carefully. When the staple is a starchy fruit, root or tuber such as yam, eddoe or plantain, it should be served with food from animals such as fish, eggs or meat. Such meals may be:

Staple	+	Food from animals
Plantain		Mackerel
Maize flour		Milk (porridge)
Potatoes		Meat stew

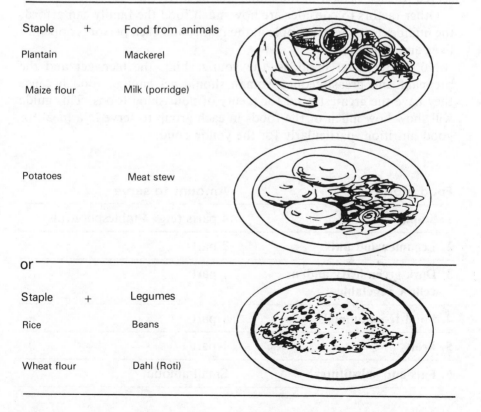

or

Staple	+	Legumes
Rice		Beans
Wheat flour		Dahl (Roti)

A meal of a starchy root or fruit staple such as yam and spinach is NOT very nourishing even when cooking oil is added. If a small amount of a protein food, eg. fish, or an egg, is added, the meal becomes more nourishing. In the same way protein foods on their own are not very satisfying.

Snacks

Snacks eaten between meals should be chosen for their nourishment as well as for taste. Good snacks are fresh fruits, milk, fruit juice, bread and egg.

How much food should be served?

How old we are, whether we are men or women and how active we usually are makes a difference in the amounts of food we need.

Babies, young children and teenagers who are growing very fast need more food than other people. Women who are pregnant or breastfeeding also need plenty of nourishing food to help their bodies work better. A person who has a lot of heavy work to do will need more food than someone who has little work to do. So the amount of food served to each person in the home will be different.

Other factors to consider are how much food the family can afford, the number and ages of people in the family and each person's appetite, likes and dislikes.

No matter what happens, the young child, the teenager and the pregnant and breastfeeding woman should get enough food because they have the greatest need for plenty of nourishing foods. This guide will show how much of the foods in each group to serve in a meal for good nutrition, particularly for the young child.

Food group	Amount to serve
1. Staple	4 parts (e.g. 4 tablespoonfuls)
2. Legumes and nuts	2 parts
3. Dark green leafy and/or yellow vegetables	1 part
4. Food from animals	1 part
5. Fruits	1 part
6. Fats and substitutes	Small amount

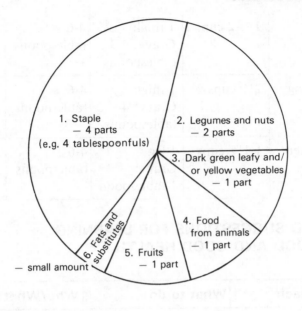

The following example will show you how to use this guide in serving a cooked meal of stewed chicken with gravy, rice and beans, pumpkin and fruit juice.

SERVING PORTIONS FOR FAMILY MEMBERS

Family Member	Meal			
	Rice and beans	Chicken	Pumpkin	Fruit juice
Young child 1-2 years	4-6 tablespoons	1 tablespoon Gravy: 1 tablespoon	1 tablespoon	½ glass
16-yr old boy or hard-working father	2-3 cups	½ breast + 1 wing Gravy: 2-3 tablespoons	4-6 tablespoons	1 glass
16-yr old girl	1½-2 cups	1 thigh Gravy: 1-2 tablespoons	4-6 tablespoons	1 glass

Pregnant woman	1½-2 cups	1 thigh Gravy: 2-3 tablespoons	4-6 tablespoons	1 glass
Breastfeeding woman	2½ cups	1 thigh Gravy: 4 tablespoons	4-6 tablespoons	1 glass
Grandmother/ Grandfather	1-1½ cups	1 leg Gravy: 1 tablespoon	4-6 tablespoons	1 glass

IDEAS AND SUGGESTIONS FOR LEARNING ABOUT FOOD AND GOOD HEALTH

What to teach	What to do	Who/What to use
Purpose: To show how eating the right kinds and amounts of food keeps people healthy.		
Messages: — Foods provide nourishment	Show how a car which runs on gas or petrol can be compared to the body which runs on the nourishment it gets from food.	
— Everyone needs nourishment to keep healthy.	Compare a baby's growth with that of an older person and show that babies need more food in relation to their size because they are growing fast.	Real foods
— The amount of food needed to provide nourishment depends on age, sex, activity, special conditions like being pregnant and growing fast.	Explain that food portions may be larger or smaller depending on how much food family members need.	Food group charts

— Foods which provide almost the same type of nourishment are grouped together. — Food can be divided into six groups.	Compare nutritional value of foods in the different food groups. Show how a meal can be made from the cheapest foods and still be nutritious. Ask some people in the group to collect prices. Using these prices work out the cost of a meal with the group.	Pictures of foods cut from newspapers or magazines.
— The most nourishing meals are made up of foods from 3-6 groups.	Ask for examples of mixtures of foods that are usually served. Show how these may be improved, if necessary (e.g. adding carrots to a stewed beans dish).	If facilities are available, demonstrate these. Also demonstrate portion sizes.
— The method of using foods from different groups at each meal is called the principle of a balanced diet.	Plan meals using the balanced diet principle.	Food group charts/real foods

6

Buying, storing and preparing foods

What to look for when buying foods

*How to handle, store and prepare
foods properly*

*Ideas and suggestions on learning about
buying, storing and preparing foods*

**Food and Nutrition
Agriculture**

WHAT YOU SHOULD BE ABLE TO DO
AFTER STUDYING THIS CHAPTER

After studying this chapter, taking part in discussions and doing the exercises and activities, you should be able to:
— advise people on how to handle, store and prepare foods properly;
— help people to understand that food needs to be handled, stored and prepared properly for good nutrition.

WHAT TO LOOK FOR WHEN BUYING FOODS

Food often takes most of the money a family earns. Since food is expensive, it is important to buy food wisely and not to waste any, either before or after cooking.

1. Staples

(a) *Starchy roots, fruits and tubers (yam, cocoyam, plantain, potato, breadfruit)*

They should be fresh, clean, firm, without any rotting spots, cuts, bruises, sunburn, worms or sprouts. 'Deep eyes' in potatoes will need plenty of paring and 'scooping' out. This is one way of not wasting too much.

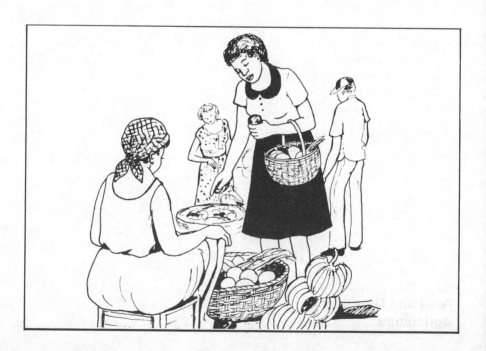

(b) *Cereals (maize, wheatflour, rice, sorghum, bread)*

If sold in clear plastic, look carefully for weevils, dirt and mould and holes in the bag. See that flour is powdery and not lumpy.

Those cereals sold in brown paper bags or clear plastic bags are usually cheaper and just as nutritious as those sold in fancy packages.

Cereals which are ready-to-eat cost much more than porridges. Cornflour and arrowroot flour cost much more than yellow maize meal and are not as nutritious.

Parboiled or brown rice, when available, is more nourishing than white rice. Much of the goodness in rice is in the brownish coating around the grains. Buy parboiled or brown rice instead of white rice.

A kilogram loaf of bread contains approximately 2/3 kg flour — bread is, therefore, much more expensive than flour. Bread is ready-to-eat and that accounts for the high price. Many other foods that are based on cereals, are expensive for a similar reason.

2. Legumes and nuts
(Cowpeas beans, groundnuts, cashews, dried coconuts)
Cowpeas and beans should be clean, sound and free from weevils, dirt, mould and mustiness. Dried cowpeas and beans are 2-3 times more nutritious for the same weight than the green ones and so are better value for money. All legumes contain about the same nourishment. As a snack, groundnuts provide much better nourishment than sweets.

Dried coconuts are fairly expensive. The 'milk' adds flavour and fat (energy) to foods. Like carrots, there is tremendous waste when the 'trash' is thrown out. Most of their nourishment is kept when they are used to make puddings, cakes or sweets like coconut 'drops'. 'Jelly' coconuts are even more expensive than the dried ones and are less nutritious. We usually drink only the water.

3. Dark green leafy/yellow vegetables
(Kale, cabbage, spinach, pumpkin, carrot)
Green leafy vegetables should be tender, crisp, bright green in colour with no decay, mould, insects, dirt or wilt. Wilted vegetables have lost some of their nourishment.

Check the weight of the food item before you buy. (A big head of cabbage could appear heavy because the leaves are loosely folded.)

Carrots should be clean, straight, free from spots and bruises and with no green showing at the top.

Carrots and pumpkin give the same nourishment. Choose whichever one is less expensive.

4. Food from animals

(a) *Milk and milk products*

Milk comes in many forms — powdered (full-cream, half-cream and skimmed), regular liquid milk in boxes and bottles, evaporated, sweetened condensed and pasteurized canned. A long-life packaged milk is now on the market in some countries.

Skimmed milk powder, sold in plastic bags, is the least expensive of all forms of milk. The fat has been removed so its energy and vitamin A value are not as high as other milks. Vitamin A is added to some types of skimmed milk powder. Skimmed milk powder should look slightly creamy, be free from lumps or caking and also smell and taste good.

Instant skimmed milk powder in fancy boxes is expensive and contains no more nourishment than the one sold in the plastic bag. It is easier to mix for drinking but the convenience costs more.

Sweetened condensed milk is used especially for the flavour it gives to certain dishes. It is just about half-sugar and does not spoil easily.

Skimmed milk powder and sweetened condensed milk are not suitable for babies.

Regular cow's milk sold in boxes usually has a date stamped on the top of the box. Look at the date. That date tells when the milk may go bad. Make sure that the one you pick up has several days to go before it may spoil. The milk boxes should not be leaking, bulging or smell sour. To save nourishment in milk which is not bought in a box use dark bottles or covered pans. Boxes, dark bottles and covered pans keep light away from the milk. Light destroys the vitamin B_2 (riboflavin) in milk.

So-called chocolate and cherry drinks are just milky drinks made of milk powder, water and sugar with cocoa powder and cherry flavouring. They do not have as much nourishment as real milk.

Goat's milk has about the same nourishment as cow's milk. The only difference is that the fat in goat's milk will not float to the top to become cream when the milk is scalded. Goat's milk is naturally homogenized which means the fat is not separated from the milk but mixed up with it.

Malted milk is made by drying ground barley malt, wheat flour and regular milk. It is used especially for flavouring and is expensive. Malted milk powder gives almost the same nourishment as wheat flour.

Cheese — Although cheese is expensive, it gives good nutrition for

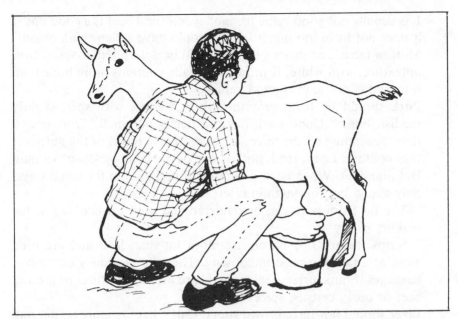

the money. Choose hard or semi-hard cheese with a rich yellow colour and tightly wrapped to keep out air. Half to one pound packets are cheaper than small wedges and slices. Most cheeses on the market are processed; they are cooked so that texture, colour and taste are different from natural cheese.

Yoghurt is a fermented milk made chiefly from skimmed milk. It is thick like custard and smooth with a slighty sour taste. Usually it is sweetened and colouring and flavouring are added. Yoghurt costs more than the same amount of milk and has no extra nourishment than the milk from which it is made.

Ice Cream is made from a liquid mix of skimmed milk and cream (butter fat or vegetable fat), sweetening and flavouring. Air is whipped in to give it a smooth texture (feel on the tongue). If sold by volume one litre should weigh just about half a kilogram.

If a litre container weighs much less than half a kilogram plenty of air has been whipped in.

(b) *Meat*

The price of meat usually depends on how the meat is cut and the part of the animal from which it comes. Liver, heart, kidney, tongue and tripe are usually lower in price than other meats and are good value for money.

Good beef should be moist, with a deep red colour, elastic and firm to the touch with solid, creamy, white fat and a good smell.

A cut of meat will be good value for money if there is more lean than fat and bone. Oxtail for example, has 45-50% waste as bone.

It is usually not good value for money. Ground beef is a good buy if it does not have too much fat. It should have a rich, pink colour. **Mutton** (goat's or sheep's flesh) should be a deep pink colour, firm in texture, with white, firm fat. It usually contains more bone than lean and is not always good value.

Pork should be firm, grayish-pink in colour, with soft, slightly reddish bones. Good pork has practically no smell. Trotters and tails, depending on the price, are expensive in terms of the nutrients they contain. Lean, fresh pork is one of the best sources of vitamin B_1 (thiamine). When pork is cured and prepared in the usual ways, only about $\frac{1}{10}$ of this vitamin is left.

The fat from pork can be rendered and used for cooking or for making pastry.

Strips (rashers) of bacon are more fat than lean and are used more as a fat than meat in cooking. They are extremely expensive. **Sausages** (Frankfurters, Salami, etc) are usually mixtures of ground beef or pork, cereals, spices and water.

Liver should not have brown spots. Calf's liver is more tender and expensive than beef liver. They provide the same nourishment.

Pork liver is grainy in texture and has a strong smell. It is extremely nutritious and is good value for money.

Rabbit should be light pink in colour, firm (somewhat like young goat's flesh, with white, creamy bones.) It is just as nutritious as chicken but more expensive. Keeping rabbits at home is more economical than buying rabbit meat in the supermarket.

(c) *Poultry (chicken, turkey, duck)*

Buying live birds may not always be cheaper than buying cleaned, plucked birds as $\frac{1}{4}$ to $\frac{1}{3}$ the weight of the live birds is feathers and intestines.

Plucked chickens are usually sold for any purpose — broiling, roasting or stewing. They should be clean, smell fresh, fleshy, with a good layer of fat, smooth, untorn skin, a good colour and no pin feathers. A larger bird has more flesh in proportion to bone than a smaller bird. A 2 kg plucked chicken is a good buy, if you can afford and store it properly. Chicken parts (legs, breasts) are very expensive when compared with the whole bird.

Stewing hens are good value for money when they are priced at about half that of the all-purpose bird. To cook them quickly, first tenderize them (by wrapping in pawpaw leaves). A bird which has just been killed takes a longer time to cook than one which has been killed 6-8 hours before cooking.

Chicken necks and backs have more food value than other 'high waste' foods, such as trotters, chicken feet, calf's heel, pig's head, pig's tail. They are usually cheaper and, therefore, good value for money.

(d) *Fish*

Fish can be bought either fresh, frozen, dried, pickled or canned. Fresh fish should have the scales lying close to the body, the flesh firm, the eyes bright and full, the gills damp and red, and·little, if any smell. Some of our 'fresh' fish is only obtainable in frozen form. The eyes are usually sunken.

Fish steaks and fillets are usually best value for money as there is no waste. Fish with the head on has a high percentage waste. Fish heads alone are usually not good value for money. They have a very high proportion of bone to flesh. Don't pay high prices for fish heads in the mistaken belief that they will 'give brains'.

Dried, smoked, salted, pickled and canned fish are good value for money. In the case of dried and smoked fish, moisture (water) is removed. Weight for weight there is more nourishment than in fresh fish.

Canned sardines and herring are good buys. High-grade salmon and tuna are expensive and contain no more food value than lower grades.

When garlic, chili, mustard or tomato sauce are added to canned fish they increase the price but do not add much food value.

(e) *Eggs*

Select eggs that are clean, free from stains and of the same size. Brown-shelled eggs have the same nourishment as white-shelled eggs. Eggs which are kept in a refrigerator or in a cool place are likely to be much fresher.

Small eggs are as good a buy as large ones if they cost at least one-fourth less. A good egg makes no sound when it is shaken. A very fresh egg has a thick, jelly-like white and a round, firm yolk.

Eggs may seem expensive but they are very nourishing and have little waste.

5. Fruits

(mango, pawpaw, orange, grapefruit, tangerine, etc)
Fresh fruits should be firm, clean and free from spots and bruises.

Don't buy fruits which are wrinkled, soft, mushy or damaged by worms or insects.

6. Fats and Substitutes

The types commonly used are cooking oil (ground nut oil, palm nut oil, soya bean oil, coconut oil, corn and soya bean oil, margarine, butter. Olive oil, suet (beef fat), lard (pork fat) are also other kinds of fats and oils. (Those that are liquid at room temperature are called oils and those that are solid are called fats.) Fats and oils should not be rancid. Butter and fortified margarine contain vitamin A. Fortified margarine is better value for money than butter. When butter and margarine become rancid the vitamin A is destroyed. Avocado (pear) is grouped among fats and substitutes and adds a fair amount of fat to the diet.

Other Foods

(a) *Sugars and sweets*

The types of sugars commonly used are granulated, brown and wet or new sugar. Sugars should be free of trash, dirt or insect parts. Brown sugar has some molasses; the smaller the amount of molasses the clearer the sugar. Granulated sugar is not as nutritious as brown sugar. Dark brown sugar is a cheap source of iron.

Molasses (a by-product of the sugar cane industry) is sold by some stores and supermarkets. It is a nutritious food and should be used when it is not too expensive. It is often a cheap source of iron. It may be used in lemonade (not as a sweetener because the amount required may cause the drink to taste bad), stewed peas, puddings, cake or had straight from the spoon.

Syrups usually fruit-flavoured, are expensive sweeteners and provide only energy. They do add flavour and colour in food preparation. A syrup can be made at home using 1½ lbs. of sugar to a pint (½ litre) of water and boiling for a short period. Add a tablespoon (15 ml) lime juice and a small amount of colouring and flavouring.

Glucose is not as sweet as cane sugar. It is easily digested and so provides energy quickly. It is very expensive.

> **Glucose should not be used instead of brown sugar in young child feeding.**

Honey provides quick energy because the sugars are easily digested. It should be in liquid form and free of gas bubbles, dirt, grit and trash. As a rule, the lighter the honey, the milder the flavour. If honey becomes solid, place it over warm water to make it liquid. Honey is expensive. However people who rear bees could use some of the honey they produce.

(b) *Sauces*

Ketchup, soya and other sauces are expensive, so they should be used in small amounts. A small amount goes a long way. Where there are cooking tomatoes to colour foods you do not need to use these sauces. Make good use of country pepper and seasoning. The powdered seasonings are usually mixed with salt and are more salt than seasoning. They are expensive.

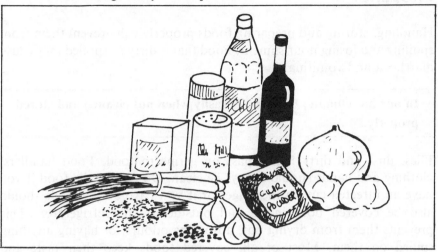

(c) *Beverages*

Mixes for hot chocolate and cocoa and chocolate-flavoured beverage powders are expensive for the nutrients they contain. They are not 'tonics' despite what the manufacturers may say. Plain milk flavoured with cocoa powder and sweetened has the same food value. It is the milk in which they are usually mixed that provides the nourishment needed by the body. Plain cocoa powder packaged in a simple plastic bag and retailed over the counter is best value for money.

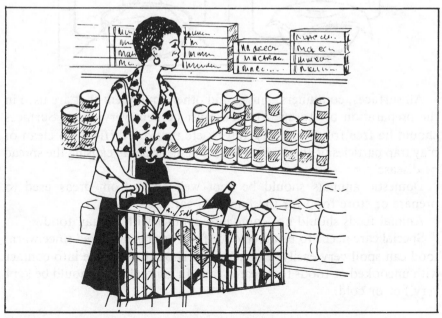

HOW TO HANDLE, STORE AND PREPARE FOODS PROPERLY

Handling, storing and preparing foods properly will prevent them from spoiling and losing nourishment. Food that is dirty or spoiled may cause diarrhoea and vomiting.

In our hot climate, food spoils easily when not cleaned and stored properly.

Flies, dust and dirty hands pass on germs to food. Food handlers' clothing and hands should always be clean. Do not handle food if you have an infected cut on the finger or if you have boils. Foods should also be covered both inside and outside of the refrigerator. This prevents them from drying out, absorbing odours, or having anything spilled on them. Most of all, covered foods keep their taste and nourishment. Foods left on a table or counter should also be covered to prevent contamination by flies.

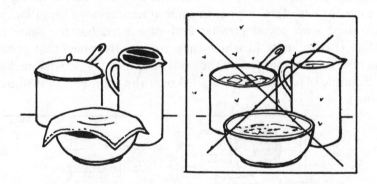

All surfaces, containers, knives and other equipment that are used in the preparation or storage of food must be kept very clean. Surfaces should be free from cracks, grooves, etc that are difficult to clean or may trap particles of food which attract pests or decay causing the spread of disease.

Domestic animals should be kept well away from areas used to prepare or store food for the family to eat.

Animal feeds should not come into contact with human food.

Special care needs to be taken once food has been cooked since warm food can spoil very easily. Cooked food should not come into contact with uncooked or foods to be eaten raw. In general food should be kept very hot or cold.

SOME IDEAS ON MAKING FOOD SAFE AND SAVING NOURISHMENT

Type of food	How to handle and store	How to prepare/use
STAPLES — starchy fruits, roots and tubers (yams, potatoes, cassava, plantain breadfruit)	Reap carefully-do not bruise or cut skins. Clean off any earth. Do not wash until ready to use. Store in a cool place in baskets or on slatted or meshed shelves where air can get around. Do not allow to sprout. Keep tubers in the dark to prevent sprouting.	Scrub skins well to remove dirt from potatoes and some types of yams. Peel them thinly, cut in pieces of the same size. Cook in small amount of boiling water. Bake or boil them in the skin. Slice them thinly and fry in hot fat to make chips.
Cereals (maize meal rice, flour, bread, biscuits)	Keep cereals like flour and maize meal dry in clean, covered containers. Store baked products in a cool, dry place to prevent mould. Store biscuits by themselves in a tightly covered pan to keep them crisp. Biscuits and bread should be stored separately. If stored with bread, biscuits absorb the moisture from the bread and become soft.	Do not wash packaged rice. Washing wastes some of the nourishment. Cook 1 part of rice in 2 parts water until all the liquid is absorbed and the grains are tender. Butter/margarine may be added to help prevent the grains from sticking together. If rice is cooked in large amounts of water, use the water poured off in soup. Do not remove the crust from bread as this is also nourishing. Removing the crust wastes good food value.
LEGUMES AND NUTS — cowpeas, beans, groundnuts	Reap groundnuts carefully so that the shells do not break. Clean and dry very well before storing. Clean peas and beans to remove dirt and grit. Store in clean, dry	Soak dried cowpeas and beans overnight or for 4-6 hours to shorten cooking time. Use the same soaking water to cook peas. Do not use baking soda to tenderize them. (Soda

Type of food	How to handle and store	How to prepare/use
	jars/pans with tight covers. Small amounts of beans can be stored in plastic bags in the refrigerator. Rub dried peas with cooking oil — (1 tablespoon to a kilogram mix with clean, dry ash before storing).	destroys B vitamins.)
VEGETABLES — dark green leafy vegetables (spinach, cabbage)	Reap or buy leafy vegetables early morning or later afternoon. Try to pick or buy when needed and avoid storing. If you must store, keep cool by placing stems in water and covering leaves in cocoyam leaf, dampened paper, cloth, or banana leaf. Place in plastic bags in refrigerator, if possible. Do not allow cabbage, string beans and cucumber to get wet before storing. They will rot faster.	When ready to cook, clean well in plenty of water before chopping. Do not let them soak in water or add baking soda to the water in which they will be soaked or cooked. Cook in a small amount of water until just tender and still bright green. Eat immediately. Do not keep hot or re-heat as vitamins are lost and colour changes. Use cooking water to make gravy or soup. Chop salad vegetables like cabbage or lettuce just before using.
Yellow Vegetables (carrots, pumpkin)	Store in a cool place or in plastic bag in refrigerator to prevent shrivelling. Save melon and pumpkin seeds — they are very nutritious. Wash and dry seeds well. Store in a container with a tight fitting lid.	Peel pumpkin thinly or cook in the skin. Cook in just enough boiling water to make tender or add to stews and soups. Scrub carrots and scrape or peel very thinly. Use carrot 'trash' in soup, gravy, pudding or seasoned rice. Use dried pumpkin seeds as snacks.

FRUITS — citrus, guava, pawpaw, mango	Reap or buy fresh and handle carefully to prevent bruising. Store citrus in a refrigerator or a cool place in baskets where air can get around the fruits. Freeze fruits and juices when in season and plentiful.	Do not allow fruits to sit around uncovered for a long time. They lose nourishment. Eat citrus pulp to get the most nourishment.
FOOD FROM ANIMALS — meat, poultry, milk, cheese, eggs	Keep cool and covered until ready to use. Do not chop raw meat, chicken or fish on the same board or counter which you use for cutting bread or chopping fruits and vegetables which will be eaten raw. Wash hands and chopping board well after handling raw meats, fish and chicken. Even if you have a refrigerator, use ground meat and organ meats the same day you buy them, unless they are frozen.	Do not wash, but wipe meats/liver with vinegar or lime juice before cooking. Thaw frozen meats slowly by leaving in the kitchen in a covered vessel or at the bottom of the refrigerator. (Use the juice ('bloody water') from the thawed meat or liver in the cooking. Do not brown meat over a high flame as this causes the meat to shrink, become tough, take longer to cook and lose nutrients. Brown the meat by adding a little burnt sugar or parched flour. Tenderize tough meats by wrapping them in pawpaw leaves or add chopped, green pawpaw to the seasoned meat and keep for an hour or two before cooking. Cook meats until just tender. Cook liver for only 8-10 minutes. The longer you cook liver the tougher it gets.

Type of food	How to handle and store	How to prepare/use
Fish	Use fresh fish quickly the same day as you buy it, or freeze it. To remove 'fishy' smell from hands, knives, sinks or bowls, rub with salt, vinegar or lime juice.	Fish is tender and cooks very quickly.
Milk	Carry and store fresh milk in dark bottles or covered pans to keep out light. Light destroys riboflavin (vitamin B_2) the main vitamin in milk. Keep pasteurized milk chilled. Keep powdered milk in air-tight jars or cans to prevent it from becoming lumpy.	Scald and cool fresh milk quickly. Keep covered. There is no need to scald pasteurized milk. Mix powdered milk by putting 1 cup powder in 4 cups water and beating well with a fork. To make a glass of milk add 2 tablespoons powder to a glass of water and beat.
Eggs	Clean eggs well. Store in a cool place away from strong smelling seasoning.	Cook slowly until tender. When properly cooked the white should be soft and jelly-like. For hard-boiled eggs place in a small pot with water and cover. Bring to the boil and continue boiling for 7-10 minutes. Cool quickly by putting in cold water.
Cheese	Keep in wrapper in which it was bought. Place in covered dish and keep cool. When cheese becomes rancid vitamin A is lost.	Lightly scrape away mould if any. Cheese can be sliced or grated and added to young child's food, made into sandwiches or sprinkled on cooked vegetables.

Buying, Storing and Preparing Foods 73

Type of food	How to handle and store	How to prepare/use
FATS AND SUBSTITUTES — butter and margarine	Place butter in dish. Cover with clean cloth. Place this dish in a larger one containing water. (Ends of cloth should be in water.) This will keep the butter cool and keep out air which will make the butter rancid. When butter becomes rancid vitamin A is lost. Keep margarine in container in which it was bought and away from strong seasoning.	

IDEAS AND SUGGESTIONS FOR LEARNING ABOUT BUYING, STORING AND PREPARING FOODS

What to teach	What to do	Who/What to use
Purpose: To show how to buy, store, handle and prepare foods properly to get the best value for money and good nutrition.	Get group members involved in checking prices, comparing costs, etc.	Real foods, particularly from group members' home gardens and the market.
Messages: When shopping for food items look at them, handle them and check weights and prices carefully before buying.	Go to the market with some members of the group and discuss food values and prices while shopping. Compare prices of foods.	Real Foods Food pages from the newspapers.
The condition in which food is bought, stored and prepared can affect the nourishment we get from it.	Show how to keep empty cans clean, dry and air-tight for storing foods.	Empty cans/packages ('mini-supermarket'). Pictures to show proper storage of foods.
Buying food in simple plastic or paper bags is cheaper than buying in fancy packages.	Ask group members to share their money-saving ideas when food shopping. Discuss 'good buys'.	Real foods, emphasizing that those that are 'good buys' in each food group can vary according to season/time of year, or availability.
— Foods which are in the same food groups are usually the same in food value. When planning meals, use the cheapest instead of the most expensive foods in any one group.	When possible, encourage home gardens, or community gardens. Show how this can save money if neighbours exchange some of the foods they grow.	Home garden, grown in cans, oil drums or car tyres.

What to teach	What to do	Who/What to use
— Buy foods that are nutritious and have little or no waste (e.g. dry fish or skimmed milk powder.)	Demonstrate how food can be prepared with the minimum of waste.	Kitchen equipment and utensils.
— Preparing foods properly will save nourishment and make them appetising.	Show the group how to prepare some foods. Let everyone taste and get the group involved in discussing how they prepare foods. Compliment for good preparation and show how poor methods could be improved.	Real foods. Examples of cooked meals.
— Don't let flashy food ads push you into buying items you don't need such as non-nutritious drink bases.	Let people give examples of foods they buy because they heard or saw them advertised. Discuss the food value and cost of these items and suggest cheaper, more nourishing substitutes.	Advertising copy from radio or T.V. (recorded on to cassette or video tape), cutouts from newspaper food advertisements or examples of ads posted in supermarkets, drug stores, etc. Consumer Educator, Nutritionist, Nutrition Assistant

7

Nutrition during pregnancy and breastfeeding

Weight gain in pregnancy

Preventing anaemia in pregnancy

Common problems which may affect nutrition during pregnancy

How to identify pregnant women who need special help

Ideas and suggestions for learning about nutrition during pregnancy and breastfeeding

Health
Food and Nutrition

WHAT YOU SHOULD BE ABLE TO DO
AFTER STUDYING THIS CHAPTER

After studying this Chapter, taking part in discussions and doing the exercises and activities, you should be able to:
— explain to mothers what to eat during pregnancy and breastfeeding;
— help mothers to become aware of the problems which may affect nutrition during pregnancy;
— explain to mothers how to deal with these problems;
— know how to help malnourished pregnant women;
— advise pregnant women about gaining weight;
— Show women how to prevent or treat anaemia during pregnancy;
— explain to fathers the importance of well-spaced pregnancies for their wives/partners.

Weight gain in pregnancy

Pregnancy is an important time in a woman's life. This is when a baby grows inside her body. To grow properly this unborn child needs a healthy and well-nourished mother.

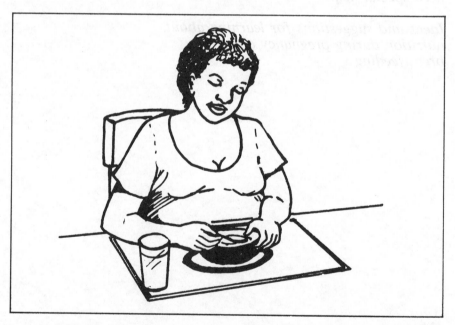

A mother-to-be needs to gain weight during pregnancy to nourish her growing baby. Women who do not gain enough weight often have babies that weigh too little. A baby that weighs less than 5½ lbs (2½ kg) is more likely to have both physical and mental problems. It may not grow normally. It may suffer more from infections and malnutrition than babies of normal weight.

A woman should gain at least 24 lbs. (11 kg) during pregnancy. The baby accounts for only part of the weight gain. Her own body must add blood, muscle, fluids and tissue which are needed for the baby's development. If she gains less than 24 lbs., the baby's chances for health and survival go down.

Weight a woman gains during pregnancy goes towards:

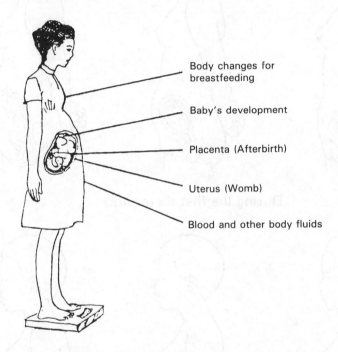

Body changes for breastfeeding

Baby's development

Placenta (Afterbirth)

Uterus (Womb)

Blood and other body fluids

If a mother is overweight, she still needs to gain for the baby's health. She should not try to lose weight while she is pregnant but should wait until after the baby is born and after breastfeeding.

When should the woman gain weight?
When and how fast the woman gains weight is just as important as the amount which she gains. A pregnant woman should gain weight smoothly and steadily. If her weight jumps suddenly, she should see the doctor.

During the first three months, she should expect to gain about 1-2 kg. During the last six months, she needs to gain about ½ kg each week.

If she has already gained 11 kg after six or seven months of pregnancy she should continue to gain moderately until delivery. The baby puts on most of its weight during those last few months.

How the body changes as the baby develops*

During the first six months

During the last three months

* Adapted from drawings by Marcia L. Williams from "The Universal Childbirth Picture Book" by Fran P. Hosken. Lexington, Mass., Women's International Network News, 1981.

What to eat

A pregnant or breastfeeding woman needs extra good foods, especially those that are good sources of iron. She should eat a well-balanced diet containing a mixture of foods. She does not need to buy any special or high-priced foods for good nutrition. She can get the extra foods she needs by eating a little more if her ordinary meals are good and well balanced.

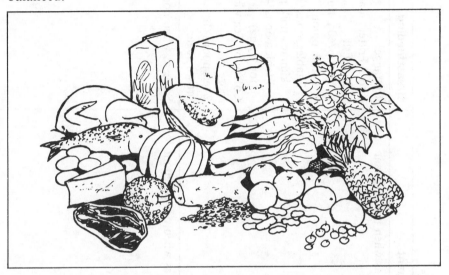

This extra food does not have to be eaten at every meal during the day. She can increase the amount of nourishment she gets at one or two meals.

PREVENTING ANAEMIA IN PREGNANCY

Some women feel weak and tired when they are pregnant. They may be anaemic. If they are anaemic, they may have difficulty in pregnancy and childbirth. Babies of anaemic mothers may be born without the 3 to 6 months' supply of iron that a normal, healthy, full-sized baby should have. An anaemic mother's breast milk may not have enough iron.

A pregnant or breastfeeding woman should have enough iron to keep herself and her baby healthy. She should eat foods that have plenty of iron every day. An acid or sour fruit drink with meals helps the body to use the iron well.

How can you tell if a woman is anaemic? It is hard to be really sure unless the blood is checked. If you look at the inside of the lips or lower eyelids, they may be pale, light pink or white. These parts should normally look bright pink.

A day's meals for a woman

Meal	Not pregnant	Pregnant	Breastfeeding
Breakfast	1 Orange 3 to 4 Fritters made from: 30 g fish ½ cup/50 g flour 1 stalk onion 2 tablespoons/15 g skimmed milk powder 2 tablespoons/30 g oil (for frying) Coffee or Tea with not more than 1 teaspoon/5 g dark brown sugar	Same as when not pregnant	1 Orange 4 to 5 Fritters made from: 30 g fish ¾ cup/60 g flour 1 stalk onion 2 tablespoons/15 g skimmed milk powder 3 tablespoons/45 g oil (for frying) Coffee or Tea with not more than 2 teaspoons/10 g dark brown sugar
Dinner (noon or evening)	Stewed Beans with Minced meat made from: ¼ cup/50 g beans 2 oz/50 g minced meat 1 tablespoon/15 g oil 2 oz/60 g Yam or potato 2 oz/60 g Ripe Plantain ½ cup/100 g Pumpkin 1 glass Lemonade (2 tablespoons/30 g dark brown sugar)	Same as when not pregnant	Same as when not pregnant

Supper (lunch)	Rice stew made from: 1/3 cup/50 g rice 50 g chicken gizzards/liver 1 cup/60 g chopped cabbage 1 tablespoon/15 g margarine 60 g Sweet Potato Pudding 1 glass Guava Juice (2 tablespoons/30 g dark brown sugar)	Rice stew made from: 1/2 cup/60 g rice 50 g chicken gizzards/liver 1 cup/60 g chopped cabbage 2 tablespoons/30 g margarine Same as when not pregnant Same as when not pregnant	Same as when pregnant
Snack		1 small packet/30 g groundnuts	Same as when pregnant
Total Calories (Energy) for the Day	2,100	2,400	2,600

A pregnant women should eat meals which contain iron-rich foods

Some of the foods which have plenty of iron are:
— beans and legumes, especially dried;
— dark green leafy vegetables;
— liver, kidney, heart;

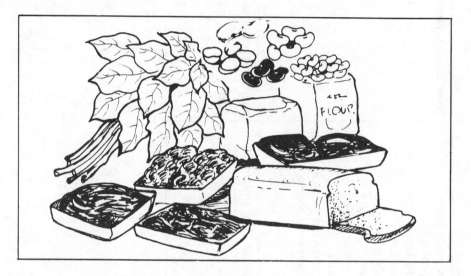

— dark brown sugar, sugar;
— sugar cane juice and molasses.
Iron is added to wheat flour; so bread has some iron.

A pregnant woman should visit the doctor, Clinic or Health Centre by at least the 4th month of her pregnancy.

At the clinic the pregnant woman's blood will be checked. She will be given iron pills, or pills which contain both iron and folate (a B vitamin) to build strong blood for her and her baby. Remind the mother to follow directions for taking the iron tablets. It's a good idea for her to take the tablets right after a main meal.

She should not take the iron tablets with tea (the one sold in the shop), coffee and milk. These prevent the body from using the iron properly. Milk provides good nourishment for a pregnant or breast-feeding woman, so it is a good drink. If the woman tell you that the iron tablets upset her, or cause side effects, encourage her to talk the problem over with her nurse or doctor. They may give her another type of iron. Remind her not to stop taking the iron as her body needs it especially at this time, and later during breastfeeding.

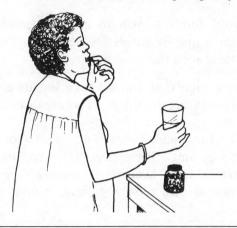

> **Remember...**
> It costs very little more to provide the extra food needed during pregnancy. The cost of the extra foods for breastfeeding is much less than the costs of canned feeds, bottles and teats.
> If the mother is already eating well, she should just eat a little more of the foods she enjoys such as:
> — yam, plantain, flour, rice and bread
> — dried peas and beans
> — mackerel, sardines, tilapia
> — skimmed milk powder and cheese
> — dark brown sugar, molasses
> — spinach, cabbage, kale
> — kidney, heart and liver.

> **All pregnant women should take iron tablets.**

COMMON PROBLEMS WHICH MAY AFFECT NUTRITION DURING PREGNANCY

Problem	How to deal with it
'Morning Sickness' (Nausea, Vomiting)	Eat a light, sweet meal before going to bed at night, e.g. a glass of milk with sugar and biscuits. Have dry bread or biscuits before getting out of bed in the morning. Eat small amounts of foods at frequent intervals — eat 5 or 6 meals a day. Drink fluids between, rather than with meals. Avoid greasy and fried foods.

Heart burn	Avoid foods known to cause discomfort. Use an antacid only if absolutely necessary. Don't take the antacid with the iron tablets.
Constipation	Drink plenty of fluids. Take liquids early morning before eating anything. This often causes the bowels to move. Eat fruits and foods with fibre (roughage), e.g. cabbage and other greens, unrefined maize meal. Take a mild laxative if necessary, e.g. Milk of Magnesia. Exercise regularly. Home gardening is good.

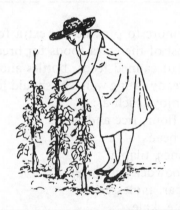

How to identify pregnant women who need special help

1. Women from poor families who are unemployed with no land, etc.
2. Women who are widows or have been deserted by their partners and have no type of family support.
3. Mothers who have given birth to many babies over a short time.
4. Women who are ill from diseases like tuberculosis.
5. Women who look thin, meagre and depressed.
6. Mothers whose previous babies have been small and malnourished.
7. Teenagers.
8. Women with babies dying in their first year of life.
9. Mothers who are overburdened with work inside or outside the home.
10. Women who are very worried about becoming a mother particularly for the first time.

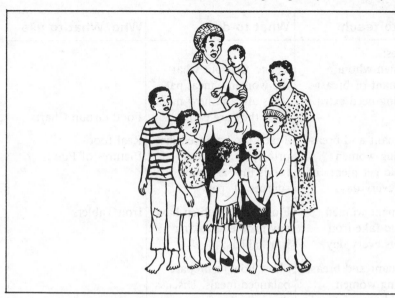

All these women need extra help. This is what you can do:

— Visit them often.
— Encourage them to eat as good a mixture of foods as they can afford.
— Let them be the first ones to receive iron or food supplements when available.
— Help them to get proper health care.
— Encourage other members of the household to do some of the house and field work and lessen the burden of work on the woman.

IDEAS AND SUGGESTIONS FOR LEARNING ABOUT NUTRITION DURING PREGNANCY AND BREASTFEEDING

What to teach	What to do	Who/What to use
Purpose: To show that it is important for a woman to eat properly when she is pregnant or breastfeeding and how this can be done.		

What to teach	What to do	Who/What to use
Messages: — Women who are pregnant or breast-feeding need extra food.	Try to find out what the women's meal patterns are and how much food they are eating.	Food Group Charts
— Pregnant and breast-feeding women should get plenty of iron every day.	Teach the balanced diet principle. Show real foods that are good sources of iron.	Real foods Pictures of Foods
— Pregnant women should take iron tablets every day.	Find out if women have any problems taking iron tablets.	Iron Tablets
— Pregnant and breast-feeding women should eat mixtures of foods from different groups.	Show how to prepare balanced meals. Discuss the amount of extra food pregnant and breastfeeding women should eat. Plan a special lunch or dinner to which the babies' father could be invited.	
— Pregnant women should gain weight during pregnancy.	Have the pregnant women in the group weigh themselves, then discuss their weight gain.	Scale
— Pregnant women who are not well-nourished are more likely to have small babies who are not properly developed, than women who are well-nourished.	Discuss how their diets can be improved. Questions to start discussion: What kinds of food should a pregnant woman eat? How much should a pregnant women eat and why? Why is it important for a pregnant women to eat the right kinds of foods?	Samples of meals. Real foods. Pictures of foods with plenty of iron.

8

Breast feeding

Why 'breast is best'

Helping mothers to breastfeed successfully

Expressing and storing breastmilk

Why bottlefeeding is bad

Situations that need special attention

Ideas and suggestions for learning about breastfeeding

Health
Food and Nutrition

WHAT YOU SHOULD BE ABLE TO DO
AFTER STUDYING THIS CHAPTER

After studying this chapter, taking part is discussions and doing the exercises and activities, you should be able to:
— explain that breastfeeding is the best, most natural and safest way to feed a baby;
— show a mother how to breastfeed;
— explain why bottlefeeding is bad;
— show a mother how to deal with any difficulties she may have with breastfeeding.

WHY 'BREAST IS BEST'

If all babies are to be healthy and grow well, they must be fed breast milk.

Milk comes from the breast even before the baby is born. When baby suckles at the nipple, this causes the milk to come into the breast and continue to flow.

Breast milk contains all the nourishment a healthy baby needs. It is a food produced by the mother's body especially for the baby. Breast milk also has substances which protect the baby from getting running belly or other infections which make baby sick.

When the mother breastfeeds and holds her baby close she gives warmth and security, as well as food. This makes mother and baby close and loving.

Breastfeeding often, and without giving baby any other kind of milk can prevent a woman from getting pregnant. To be fully protected, the couple should use a contraceptive method which does not affect breastfeeding.

Advantages of breastfeeding

Breast milk goes straight from the mother to the baby and never gets too hot or too cold.

Human milk is different from cow's milk and formula. It contains just the right amount and type of nourishment for human babies.

If a mother breastfeeds, she loses the weight put on during pregnancy more quickly than if she does not. The womb will get smaller faster when a mother breastfeeds.

Breast milk does not give baby an upset stomach or a rash or make him constipated.

Breastfeeding is an ideal way for a mother to show love and

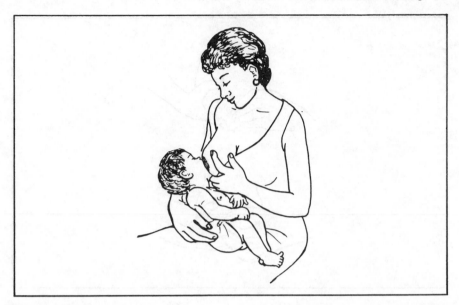

tenderness towards her baby. It helps her to know her baby well. It makes mother and baby close to each other while breastfeeding and afterwards. Breastfeeding makes a baby feel safe, contented and loved.

The mother who breastfeeds will not have to use a feeding bottle or buy cans of baby feed. It costs much less for the mother to eat a little more than to buy special foods for the baby. Eating extra food gives her energy to make breast milk. Breastfeeding also saves time as the mother will not have to mix baby feeds.

HELPING MOTHERS TO BREASTFEED SUCCESSFULLY

Breastfeeding is the natural way for a mother to feed her baby. She must be relaxed, contented and well prepared to feed her baby well.

Before baby is born
When a mother is pregnant, her breasts get bigger. She should support them with a well fitting, sturdy bra, made of cotton.

Take care of the breasts
She should wash her breasts every day and make sure she dries them well. She should rub the nipples with vaseline, lotion, cream or oil to keep them soft. She should also pull the nipples out a few times so that they will stand out. If the mother does this every day, her nipples will not become sore when she is breastfeeding baby. A good time to do this is when she is taking her daily bath.

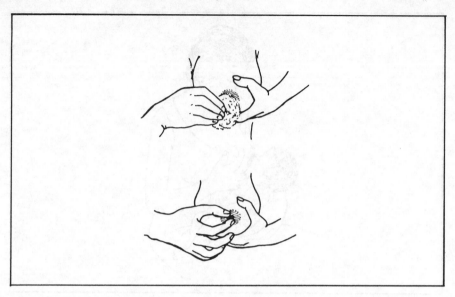

Colostrum

A pregnant woman may notice a thin, yellowish fluid coming from the nipples. This is called colostrum. At about six weeks before the baby is due, she should squeeze some of this from her breasts every day. This will help her milk flow more easily after baby is born.

When baby is born

A new-born baby should be put to the mother's breast as soon as possible. Baby should suck on each breast for 3-4 minutes. The baby will swallow some of the thin yellowish fluid — the colostrum — and

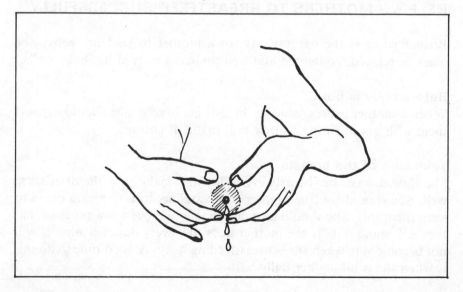

this will nourish the baby until the milk 'comes in'. The colostrum will also protect the baby from some germs and diseases. Colostrum, baby's first food, is all the new-born baby needs.

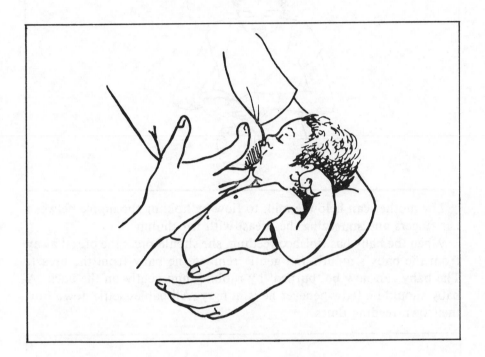

How to breastfeed baby

When she is breastfeeding, the mother should be comfortable. The baby's head and back should be supported with her arm. The nipple, and as much as possible of the dark area around it, should be put into the baby's mouth. If baby sucks on the nipple alone, he will not get enough milk and the nipple may become sore.

The breast must be held from the baby's nose with the second or third finger of his mother's hand. If the breast rests on the baby's nose, he will not be able to breathe properly. Baby should feed for 10-15 minutes on each breast.

If the baby falls asleep before he has finished feeding, the mother should flick the soles of his feet or tap his chin so that he sucks hard. The more baby sucks, the more milk is produced. After baby has finished breastfeeding, both breasts should be empty. If they still feel full after feeding, the mother should squeeze some milk from each breast.

When the baby is ready for the next feed, the breasts will be quite full again. Baby should begin feeding at the breast suckled last.

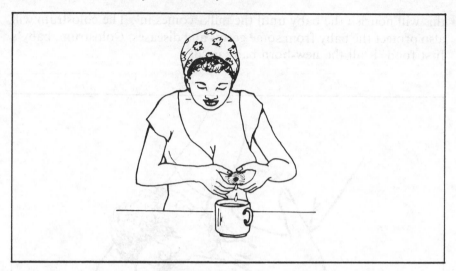

The mother can help the milk to flow by holding the nipple between her fingers and squeezing the breast with her thumb.

When the baby has finished feeding, she should press the breast away from the baby's mouth and gently remove the baby from the breast. The baby can now be 'burped' by rubbing him gently on the back. A baby should be fed whenever he is hungry. All babies settle down into their own feeding times.

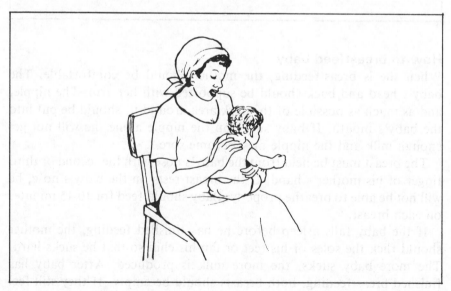

A mother who is relaxed and contented will be able to breastfeed her baby better than one who is worried and tense. Any kind of worry can slow down the flow of milk. Family members can help with the housework or with caring for younger children so that she can relax and the baby can get plenty of milk from the breast.

A mother may find it hard to breastfeed if she:

1. is young
2. has never breastfed before
3. has no relatives or friends to encourage and help her
4. has other young children
5. is expected to work soon after the baby is born.

EXPRESSING AND STORING BREASTMILK

A breastfeeding mother can squeeze out the milk from her breasts if they are still full after feeding and if she feels uncomfortable. Squeezing out milk from the breast is called 'expressing'. If mother has to leave her baby for several hours she can also express her breast milk so that the baby can continue getting breast milk while she is away.

The baby should be fed the expressed breastmilk from a clean cup and spoon.

How to express breastmilk

1. A mother should wash her hands, breasts and nipples and have ready clean container to collect the milk. A wide-mouthed jar with a cover could be used. Bottle and cover should be sterilized (by boiling 10-15 minutes) before using.
2. She should find a quiet spot where she can be alone.
3. She should gently massage the breast with one hand all over, starting from the top and working downwards.
4. She should support the breast with the other hand from underneath, with the thumb resting on top of the dark area around the nipple.
5. She should press this area gently with the thumb. The milk will begin to flow.
6. The milk should be collected in the container and stored. If available, a refrigerator should be used to store the milk for no more than 12 hours. Expressed breast milk can also be frozen, thawed and used for feeding.

Store thawed milk in a refrigerator. If a refringerator is not available the milk should be kept at room temperature for no more than two hours. After this time, it should be thrown away.

WHY BOTTLEFEEDING IS BAD

A mother should avoid bottle feeding. Bottle feeding is bad for many reasons:

1. Money has to be spent to buy feeding bottles, teats and cans of baby feed, which are very expensive.
2. A mother will have to wash and boil feeding bottles and this takes time and expensive fuel.
3. Feeding bottles and teats are hard to keep clean. Many babies get running belly (diarrhoea) from germs which grow in bottles that are not properly cleaned and boiled. Some babies get so sick that they may even die.
4. Mixing baby feeds takes a lot of time.
5. If the feed is mixed too weak, baby will starve and become malnourished.
6. If there is no stove to boil water and no refrigerator to store feeds, the milk will not be pure enough for baby and will spoil easily.

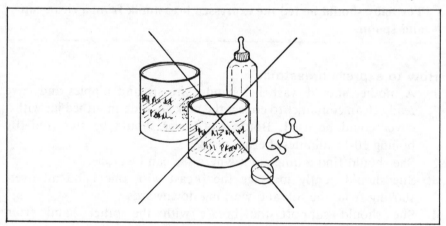

SITUATIONS THAT NEED SPECIAL ATTENTION

1. First pregnancy

The woman who is pregnant for the first time needs special teaching, support and encouragement. She needs help to breastfeed successfully and to enjoy it. Experienced mothers or other relatives, the health worker and the baby's father can all help.

Sometimes a mother does not breastfeed successfully because she is worried about many things. She may also feel that she will not be able to breastfeed. The health worker should spend plenty of time with her and the baby's father to discuss any problems.

If a mother is supposed to get maternity leave, health workers should help her get all the allowances and leave to which she is entitled. The health worker should also tell the mother about day-care centres (creches) and clinics where both mother and child can get health care. In some cases the health worker may even help to start a day-care centre and mother's group.

2. The undernourished mother

Most mothers who are poorly nourished produce rich breast milk to feed the baby. They may produce slighly less milk than well nourished mothers, but the milk will be just as nourishing and good. This milk will help ensure that the baby develops and keeps healthy during the first months of life.

> **However, it is very important that the mother gets enough to eat while she is pregnant and while she is breastfeeding.**

She should eat local foods that she knows well, that are nourishing, easy to get and not too-expensive. The health worker should advise her what to eat and show her how she can get the extra foods she needs.

If the mother is not well, the health worker should find out why. It may be that she really does not know what she should eat. Once the health worker knows what is wrong, she should guide the mother in practical ways of getting a good diet.

There are different ways of helping the mother and family get extra food. One way is to help them to work together, planting gardens and learning useful skills such as sewing and craft work, which they can use to earn extra money. If a mother does less work, particularly heavy work during pregnancy and breastfeeding, she will be able to save energy to look after herself and her child properly.

3. Mothers who have a difficult delivery

After a difficult or long labour, the mother may be too tired to breastfeed right away. But remember, the sooner the mother suckles her baby after birth, the sooner the milk will flow and breastfeeding begin. Breastfeeding should begin within the first half hour or as soon as possible after delivery.

In general, drugs should not be used during pregnancy, delivery and breastfeeding **unless they are absolutely necessary**. Drugs may interfere with breastfeeding or the composition of breast milk. If drugs are used during delivery, such as in forceps and caesarean section deliveries, every effort should be made to get breastfeeding started as soon as the mother feels well.

4. Babies that have difficulty sucking

Some babies find it difficult to feed from the breast at first. Examples of such babies are those who are tiny at birth, those born before they are due, or those who are deformed in the lip or mouth or have tetanus (lock-jaw).

Whatever the baby's condition, breast milk is still the best and most nutritious food. If the baby cannot for some reason take the breast, the mother should be encouraged to squeeze out her milk into a clean cup and feed it to her baby with a clean spoon. The breastmilk should be given to the baby right away and should not be stored for more than two hours out of a refrigerator.

Small amounts of milk squeezed from the breast and fed often to the baby will nourish and protect him from infection, just as normal breastfeeding would. As the baby grows and is able to suck or as his appetite develops, the mother should begin to breastfeed whenever he is hungry.

5. Breast problems

Very full (engorged) breasts

When the breasts are full, hard and tender, they are engorged. Engorgement of the breasts can be painful. The best way to reduce

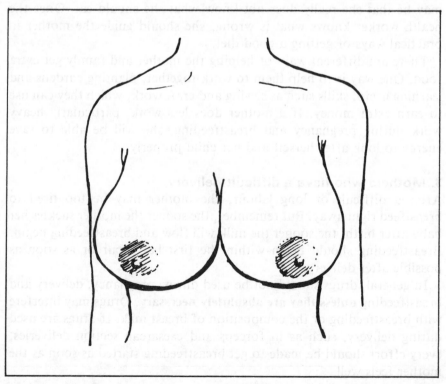

engorgement is by feeding the baby more often for shorter periods. The mother may also squeeze the milk from her breasts by hand or by breast pump and give this milk to the baby using a clean cup and spoon. The mother should be sure to wash her hands, and if a pump is used, to wash this properly before squeezing out the milk.

To squeeze out her milk by hand the mother should hold the breast with both hands and gently massage it towards the nipple. As her fingers reach the nipple area she should press down and squeeze the milk out of the nipple. The mother should repeat this four or five times. Sometimes she may feel lumpy areas which are tender. These are the glands swollen with milk. They should be softened by applying a warm compress and gently massaging them.

Breast abscess

A breast abscess may develop when the milk ducts are blocked. When this happens the breast becomes painful. The mother should be treated at the clinic. She should try to continue feeding the baby from the healthy breast.

Short or flat nipples

If the mother has short or flat nipples, before each feed she should pull out the nipple until it is long enough for the baby to hold well in the mouth. If she pulls out the nipple often during pregnancy, she should not have short nipples during breastfeeding.

When feeding the baby the mother should pull out the nipple and press the baby firmly against the breast. She should keep the baby's nose free for breathing by putting a finger between the nose and her breast. Squeezing out some of the milk will make it easier for baby to suck.

Cracked, sore nipples

Nipples can become very sore when the baby sucks very strongly. Sore nipples are painful and can cause the mother to stop breastfeeding.

To prevent the nipples from becoming sore and to help them get better if they are sore, the mother should expose the nipple to air and sunlight and feed the baby often. If the mother feeds her baby first from the breast with the less sore nipple, the baby will not have to suck so strongly at the sore nipple.

It is very important that the baby should also be held in the correct position for breastfeeding. The baby's mouth should take most of the dark portion around the nipple and not just the nipple alone. The mother should change her position, that is, sit up or lie down, so that pressure of the baby's gum will be on different parts of the nipple.

If the nipples are too painful for the mother to breastfeed, she should squeeze out her milk by hand or pump. She should then give the milk to her baby using a cup and spoon.

6. Mothers who do not have enough milk

Too little milk is a reason mothers often give for not breastfeeding or stopping breastfeeding early. In fact, the milk the mother produces is usually enough for the baby during the first 4 to 6 months of life. When the mother says she has too little milk, it often means that she does not believe that she can produce enough milk.

The mother who thinks that she is not producing enough milk during the first week needs strong encouragement to feed the baby very often. Frequent sucking at the breast will help stimulate the flow of milk. It will also help the mother gain confidence and get used to breastfeeding.

If the baby is not gaining enough weight and is very fussy, he may not be getting enough breast milk. Before recommending any other kind of feeding, the health worker should check to see if the mother is breastfeeding correctly.

> **During the prenatal period, a mother should be taught to express breast milk by hand. Other babies may need her milk; likewise, her baby may need another mother's milk.**

7. When babies have to stay in hospital

In cases where the baby needs to stay in hospital, the mother should be allowed to stay close to the baby and continue breastfeeding. The mother should also be encouraged to express her breastmilk at the hospital. Pre-term and small-for-date babies can be fed solely on expressed breastmilk, by nasogastric tube, medicine dropper or cup and spoon, until able to suckle. The community worker can encourage hospital personnel to have the mother come to the hospital often and help to get the mother to and from the hospital.

8. When a mother has to go out to work

Sometimes a mother has to return to work when her baby is 6-8 weeks old. **These babies should still get breastmilk.** About two weeks before returning to work she should get her baby used to taking expressed breast milk from a cup and spoon. She should also explain to the baby's 'caretaker' that the baby must continue getting breastmilk while she is at work. She should teach the caretaker how to feed the baby the breast milk with a cup and spoon.

When a mother starts work she should try to breastfeed the baby at least once before leaving home. She should also express enough milk for at least one feed while she is away. If she can come home during the work-day, she should breastfeed at that time. As soon as she returns from work she should breastfeed again also, and as often as the baby wants during the evening and night.

9. Breastfeeding again after stopping

If a baby is ill, whether for a short or long time, this can cause him to lose his appetite and stop breastfeeding. This does not mean that the baby cannot be breastfed again.

Even if the flow of breast milk has stopped altogether, it can be started again. (In the meantime the mother should use a cup and spoon to feed the baby some other type of milk which she can afford.)

To start breastfeeding again, the mother should let the baby suck at the breast for several minutes before giving any other food. It is the baby's sucking at the breast that encourages milk to flow.

Milk usually starts flowing again after about a week and soon the mother should be able to feed her baby from the breast again.

> **The community worker should remember that all these situations can be difficult for the mother to manage and that she may need the special advice and help of the health team.**

IDEAS AND SUGGESTIONS FOR LEARNING ABOUT BREASTFEEDING

What to teach	What to do	Who/What to use
Purpose: To describe the advantages of breastfeeding and show how to breastfeed. Messages: — Breastfeeding is the safest, cheapest and most nourishing way to feed a young baby.	Gather costs of canned baby foods, bottles and teats. Show how much money, time and effort can be saved by breastfeeding. Help mothers figure out how much they have to spend for breastfeeding. Compare to bottle feeding.	Cans of baby formula, bottles and teats, showing prices.

What to teach	What to do	Who/What to use
— Breastfeeding is natural and easy if the mother prepares for it properly while she is pregnant.	Have someone who can sew give a demonstration on how to make a maternity bra. Let those mothers who can sew, make bras for themselves and for others. (Get contributions of suitable material from local storeowners or other sources.)	Sewing Instructor/ Seamstress/Home Economics Instructor.
— Eating wisely while breastfeeding is necessary for the good health of baby and mother. No special foods are needed, just a well-balanced diet of different foods	Plan meals for a breast-feeding mother.	Food Groups Chart Real Foods
— Baby should be put to the breast as soon after birth as possible. Colostrum provides nourishment and protection for the baby.	Group discussion of false views and attitudes towards breastfeeding.	Public Health Nurse
— To breastfeed successfully mothers should be relaxed and know how to breastfeed.	Encourage mothers to practise caring for and preparing the breasts for breastfeeding. Bring in mothers who are breast-feeding successfully. They can talk to the group or, if willing, give an actual demonstration. Discuss advantages of breastfeeding.	Mother who are breast-feeding or have breast-fed successfully.

What to teach	What to do	Who/What to use
— Even if a mother has to return to work when baby is still very young, baby can still get breastmilk.	Show mothers how to express breastmilk. Get mothers who work to talk about the problems of breastfeeding and working. (Be sure to include some women who have done it successfully.)	Mothers who have expressed breastmilk successfully. Public Health Nurse. Breast pump, clean jars with covers; pot and water for sterilizing jars and covers.
— Bottlefeeding is bad for babies because it is expensive and germs grow easily in feeding bottles.	Show how difficult it is to keep a feeding bottle and teat clean by using examples. Questions or Discussion: How soon after birth should a mother start to breastfeed her baby? Should the baby be given the watery colostrum that comes into the breast before the milk starts flowing? Should a baby be given sugary water? For how many months should a baby be breastfed? Does breastfeeding keep a mother from getting pregnant? Why do some babies get sick with running belly?	Dirty feeding bottle and teat.

9

Young child feeding

From breast milk to mixed diet

Feeding the young child 4-6 months

Feeding the young child 7-12 months

Feeding the young child one year and over

Feeding the young child when he is sick

Recipes for making a young child's meals

Ideas and suggestions for learning about young child feeding

Health
Food and Nutrition

WHAT YOU SHOULD BE ABLE TO DO AFTER STUDYING THIS CHAPTER

After studying this chapter, taking part in discussions and doing the exercises and activities, you should be able to:
— explain to mothers/childminders that at 4 months a child needs nourishing foods in addition to breast milk;
— show mothers/childminders how to prepare foods for a baby 4-6 months old;
— advise mothers/childminders that a baby 6 months and over can eat meals cooked for the family;
— show mothers/childminders how to prepare foods for the baby 6 months and over.

FROM BREAST MILK TO MIXED DIET

A baby's first food is breast milk which is an excellent food. Breast milk alone satisfies the baby for the first four months of life. After four months, breast milk alone is not enough to make the baby grow well. Other foods need to be given in addition to breast milk. When new foods are added to the baby's diet and the breast milk given gradually becomes less, we call this 'weaning'.

The best foods for children who are being weaned are:

1. High in energy (calories)
Young children need energy. Staples, especially cereals, are good sources of energy. Foods from animals and fruits also provide energy. Fat, oil and sugar are good sources of energy. Enough of good mixtures of foods will provide the nutrients the young child needs for proper growth and development.

2. Easy to digest
The first new foods babies eat should be very soft and easy to digest. Later, as teeth grow and as the digestive system develops, more solid foods should be added.

3. Pure and clean
Baby's food should be as fresh as possible. In homes where foods cannot be kept cold very easily, baby's food must be cooked before each meal.

4. Inexpensive and easy to prepare

Many families do not have much money to spend on food. Taking out baby's share of food from the meals cooked for the family does not cost extra money. Since the young child's stomach is small, he needs feeding more often than the rest of the family. He is also growing very fast so needs nourishing food several times a day, not only at main meals.

FEEDING THE YOUNG CHILD 4 TO 6 MONTHS

1. Breastfeed
2. Give porridge and fruit juice

How to make the porridge

The porridge should be made thick and fed from a clean cup or bowl and spoon. Make porridge with maize meal, rice, or banana. Cook the baby's porridge with whole milk or add a thick paste of milk powder to the porridge after cooking. Skimmed milk powder tends to cause the porridge to burn, so add it (mixed with water) after the porridge is cooked. Any one of these kinds of milk may be used:
— cow's milk
— dried whole milk powder
— dried skimmed milk powder
— evaporated milk
— goat's milk

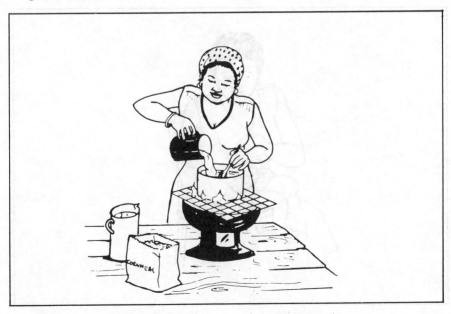

How to feed the porridge to baby

Use brown sugar to sweeten the thick porridge. This will give mainly energy as well as some iron. Condensed milk can be used to sweeten the porridge too, but brown sugar is better. Do not use too much. For more energy, add margarine.

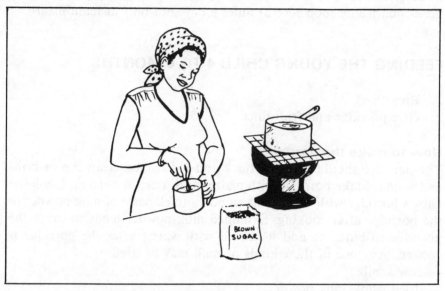

Give the baby porridge twice a day. Start with 2 or 3 teaspoons, then give more, a little at a time. When baby is six months old, he should be having ½ a cup of thick porridge twice a day.

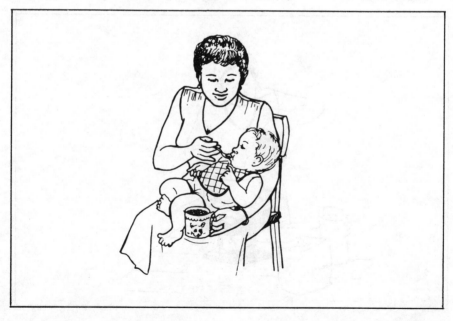

How to prepare fruit or juice

Baby can have any fruit — like mango, orange, grapefruit, guava, ripe banana. The fruit can be juiced or mashed with a fork. If the fruit is sour, sweeten it with a little brown sugar.

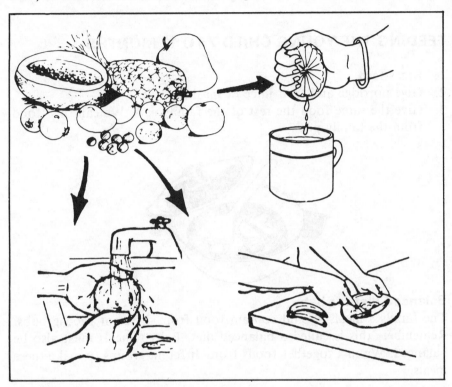

How to feed the fruit or juice to baby

Feed baby the juice or mashed fruit from a clean cup and spoon. Start with two or three teaspoons, then give more, a little at a time. By the time baby is six months old he should be having about half a cup of juice or mashed fruit every day.

Guide to feeding a 4 to 6 month old baby

Breastfeeding is still important, up to one year old or even older. If the mother has to go to work, she can still breastfeed her baby in the morning and at night. Here is what she can give the baby:

early morning	— breast milk
breakfast	— fruit juice or mashed fruit
mid-morning	— porridge
lunch	— breast milk
evening	— porridge
bedtime	— breastmilk

If the mother is at home, she should breastfeed the baby after feeding the porridge. To start porridge or any new food, give it before breastfeeding when the baby is more likely to take it because he is hungry.

FEEDING THE YOUNG CHILD 7 TO 12 MONTHS

1. Breastfeed
2. Give porridge and fruit juice or mashed fruit
3. Give the same food the rest of the family eats. We call this 'food from the family pot'.

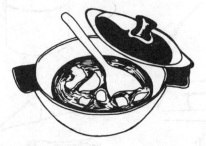

Balanced diet for baby

The family's meals should contain food from different food groups. Remember, this is called a balanced diet. Baby's meals must also be balanced. We mix together foods from different groups to make these meals:

Two food groups

Plantain + mackerel
Rice + beans

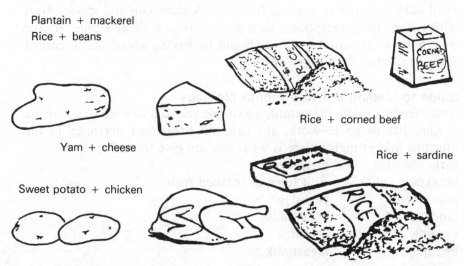

Rice + corned beef

Yam + cheese

Rice + sardine

Sweet potato + chicken

Three food groups

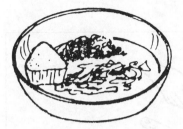 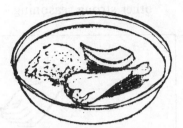

Yam + spinach + fish   Rice + pumpkin + chicken

Four food groups

Rice + beans + spinach + mutton
Yam + beans + cabbages + tripe
Yam or dumpling + beans + carrot + beef
Rice + groundnuts + pumpkin + stewed beef

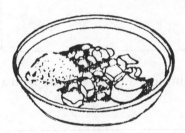

Rice + beans + spinach + mutton

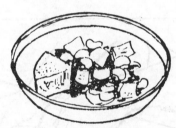

Yam + beans + cabbage + tripe

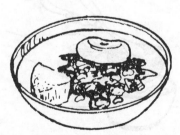

Yam or dumplings + beans + carrot + beef

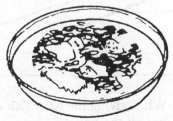

Rice + groundnuts + pumpkin + stewed beef

How to prepare baby's food from the 'family pot'

1. Take out the baby's food before adding hot pepper, curry or any other strong seasoning.

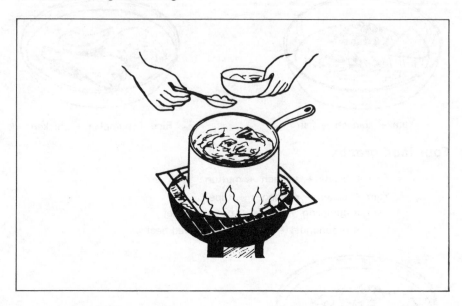

2. Mash the food with a fork or rub it through a **clean** strainer with a **clean** spoon.

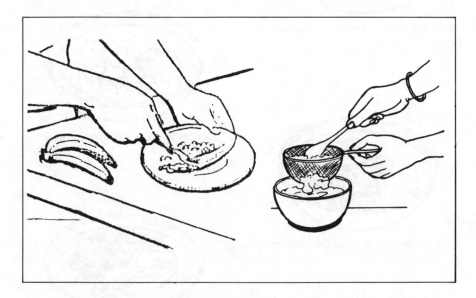

3. When giving the baby fish or meat, cut it into small pieces and take out all the bones.

4. Soften baby's food with butter or margarine or a little 'pot water' or gravy.

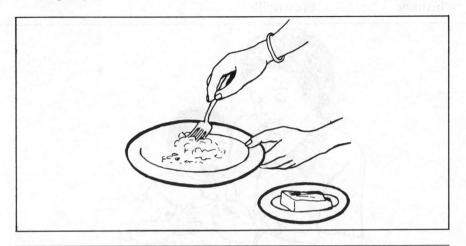

Always feed baby from a clean cup and spoon.

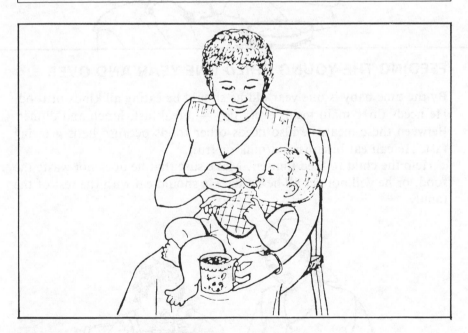

Guide to feeding a 7 to 12 month old baby

early morning	—	breast milk
breakfast	—	juice or fruit, porridge, bread and butter
mid-morning	—	biscuits and milk
lunch	—	thick porridge made with milk, maize meal and mixed with brown sugar

afternoon	—	fruit
evening	—	rice + groundnuts + pumpkin + meat
bedtime	—	breastmilk

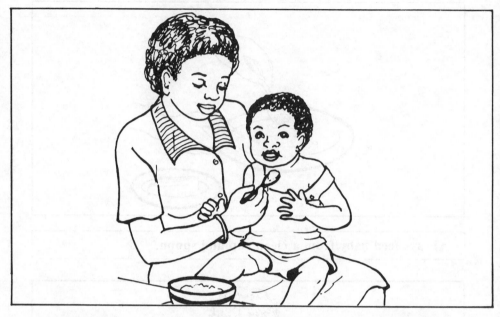

FEEDING THE YOUNG CHILD ONE YEAR AND OVER

By the time baby is one year old he should be eating all kinds of food. He needs three main meals every day — breakfast, lunch and dinner. Between these meals he also needs other foods because he is growing fast. He can eat biscuits and milk or fruit.

Help the child to feed himself. Make sure that he does not waste the food, or he will not get all he needs. He should eat with the rest of the family.

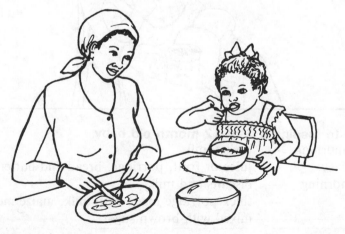

Guide to feeding a child one year and over

early morning	—	juice or fruit
breakfast	—	sardine fritter and milk
mid-morning	—	biscuits with milk
lunch	—	porridge made with milk, cereal and mixed with brown sugar
afternoon	—	fruit
evening	—	sweet potato + spinach + mackerel, lemonade
bedtime	—	milk

At 4-6 months start feeding porridge and fruit. Continue breastfeeding.

Breastfeed Baby 0-4 Months

By 1 year give family meal cut in small pieces. Continue porridge, fruit and breastfeeding.

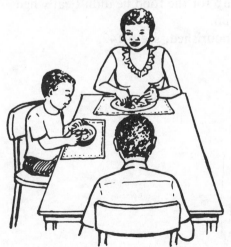

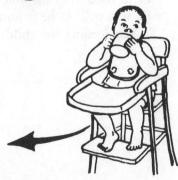

By 9 months
Give mashed foods from the family meal. Continue porridge, fruit and breastfeeding.

FEEDING THE YOUNG CHILD WHEN HE IS SICK

When a child is sick or has an infection, he needs more food than usual. The food must be more nourishing than usual so the body can fight illness. Encourage the mother not to stop giving certain foods during illness.

Milk is a good food for sick children. Breast milk is the best food for sick babies.

A mother should never stop breastfeeding when a baby is sick.

If baby cannot suck, the breast milk can be squeezed out into a clean cup and fed to baby with a spoon. If baby does not suck and the milk is not squeezed out, the milk will dry up.

For feeding the child who has diarrhoea (running belly), see pages 159-160.

Sometimes a sick child may not want to eat. The mother should try very hard to get him to eat. She should give foods which are easy to swallow like thick porridge or bread soaked in milk. She should give some yellow and orange vegetables and fruits like pawpaw and mango, soft cooked, dark, green, leafy vegetables like spinach and plenty of fluids. Sick children need plenty of tender, loving care. They need coaxing to eat.

When children have infections they need good nourishing food.

Remember, malnutrition makes infection worse and infection makes malnutrition worse.

When the child is better, feed him extra food. He should take enough extra food after his illness to make up for the food he didn't eat when he was sick. If he is hungry, feed him.

For feeding the child who is malnourished, see p.142.

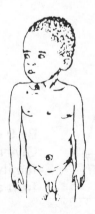

RECIPES FOR MAKING A YOUNG CHILD'S MEALS

To follow these recipes, put the spoons and cups you will use to make baby's foods up against these drawings. If you do this, you will be sure that you are using the right amounts.

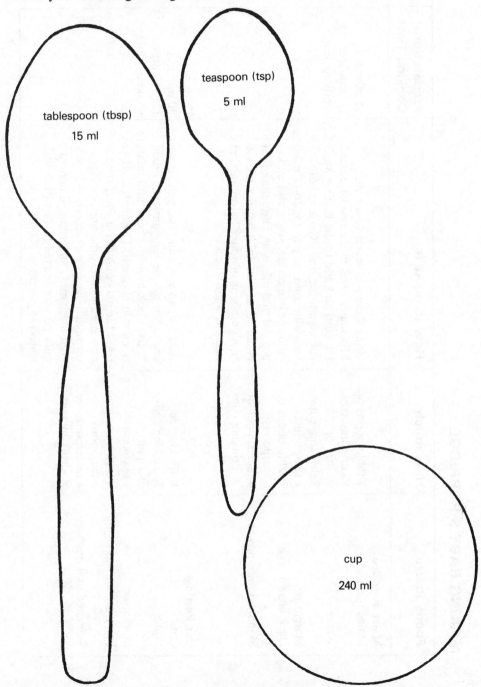

tablespoon (tbsp)

15 ml

teaspoon (tsp)

5 ml

cup

240 ml

MAKING BABY'S PORRIDGE

Foods to use	How much	How to make it	Preparation/ Cooking Time	Amount
Maize Porridge				
Maize meal	7 tablespoons or ½ drinking cup	Bring 2 cups of water to a boil. Mix maize meal in the rest of water (½ cup) and add to the boiling water, stirring all the time. Cook over low heat with cover on pan for 10-12 minutes. Add the margarine, sugar and milk powder and mix well. (You may find it easier to mix the milk powder with a small amount of water before mixing it into the maize meal	15 minutes (12 minutes (cooking time)	About 2 cups
Water	⅓ litre or 3 drinking cups			
Margarine	1 teaspoon			
Dark brown sugar	2 tablespoons or 6 teaspoons			
Skimmed milk powder	4 tablespoons or ¼ drinking cup			
Oat Porridge				
Oats	1 drinking cup	Add oats to water in saucepan. Put to cook. Stir all the time until the mixture boils. Cook over low heat until mixture is smooth about 10-12 minutes. (If you cook the oats only for a short time you may need to press the hot porridge through a sieve or strainer).	30 minutes (25 minutes cooking time)	3 drinking cups
Water	3 drinking cups or 1 pint			
Margarine	1 teaspoon			
Dark brown sugar	2 tablespoons or 6 teaspoons	Add margarine, sugar and skimmed milk powder (mixed thick with a little water) to porridge.		
Skimmed milk powder	4 tablespoons or ¼ drinking cup			

Rice Porridge				
Rice	½ drinking cup	Put the rice and cold water in a saucepan and bring to the boil. Lower the flame and simmer for 30 minutes. Press the hot porridge through a sieve or strainer and add milk powder (mixed thick with a little water), margarine and sugar to porridge.	1 hour (35 minutes cooking time)	2½ drinking cups
Water	3 drinking cups			
Skimmed milk powder	4 tablespoons or ¼ drinking cup			
Margarine	1 teaspoon			
Dark brown sugar	2 tablespoons or 6 teaspoons			
Plantain or Banana Porridge				
Peeled plantain or green banana	1-1½ medium sized bananas or ½ medium sized plantain	Grate the banana or plantain and beat in ½ cup of the water until there are no lumps. Bring the rest of the water to a boil and add the grated mixture. Stir well, turn the flame down and simmer for 15 to 20 minutes. Add the skimmed milk powder (mixed thick with a little water), margarine, dark brown sugar and cool before serving.	35 minutes (25 minutes cooking time)	About 2 cups
Water	⅓ litre or 2½ cups			
Skimmed milk powder	4 tablespoons or ¼ drinking cup			
Margarine	1 teaspoon			
Dark brown sugar	2 tablespoons or 6 teaspoons			

USING OTHER KINDS OF MILK:
1. Use cow's milk instead of water and skimmed milk powder.
2. Use only (2 cups or 2 cans) of cow's milk and add ½ cup or ½ can of coconut milk which adds flavour and fat.
3. Use ½ can of evaporated milk mixed with 1 can of water instead of cow's milk.

PREPARING BABY'S JUICES AND FRUITS

Foods to use	How much juice	How to make it	Prep. time	Amount
Juices				75 ml
Guava				
Guava pulp	1 tbsp	Cut washed guavas in halves. Scoop out pulp with a spoon. Mash and strain pulp. Add water and sugar to strained pulp and mix.	10-15 mins	50 ml
Cooled, boiled water	3 tbsp			
Dark brown sugar	1 tsp			
Grapefruit				
Grapefruit juice — freshly squeezed and strained	4 tbsp	Mix together juice, water and sugar.	10 mins	50 ml
Cooled, boiled water	2 tbsp			
Dark brown sugar	1 tsp			
Pineapple				
Pineapple, grated	¼ lb. or ½ cup	Pour water over pineapple and let it sit for 5 to 10 minutes. Rub through strainer with spoon and serve.	15-20 mins	50 ml
Cooled, boiled water	½ cup			
Orange				
	1 small or ½ large	Wash orange. Squeeze out juice. Strain and serve.	5 mins	50 ml

Mashed and strained fruit				
Guava and banana				
Guava	1 small	Wash guava and cut in half. Scoop out pulp, mash and rub through strainer. Mash banana and mix with guava.	10 mins	½ cup
Ripe banana	½ small			
Pawpaw and Orange				
Pawpaw	Small piece (50 g)	Mash pawpaw well and add orange juice. Rub through strainer and serve. You can use 1 teaspoon lime juice instead of orange.	10 mins	¼ cup
Orange juice	2 tbsp			
Pawpaw and Guava				
Pawpaw	Small piece (3 oz)	Mash pawpaw well and add guava pulp. Rub both through strainer and serve.	10-15 mins	75 ml
Guava pulp	1 tbsp			
Mango				
Mango	1 medium	Wash and peel mango. Cut flesh from seed and rub through strainer. Scrape back of strainer and mix with liquid portion.	5-8 mins	(¼ cup) 50 ml

KEY: tbsp = tablespoon   tsp = teaspoon

Remember:
As the young child gets older you can try giving him some fruits without straining them, e.g. pawpaw and mango. You may also cut some soft fruits into small pieces so that the child will learn to chew. **Be sure to take out all the seeds.**

MAKING BABY'S DINNERS

Foods to use	How much	How to make	Prep. cooking time	Amount
Rice + beans + pumpkin + chicken Cooked Rice + beans. Cooked Pumpkin Cooked Chicken Gravy	4-6 tbsp 1 tbsp 1 tbsp 1 tbsp	Remove child's portion from family pot. Cut chicken in small pieces, mix with rice and peas and pumpkin and add gravy.	5 min	6-8 tbsp (Child's portion 6-8 tbsp)
Sardine fritters Sardine Flour Tomato Water Fat	3¼ oz 1 cup 2-3 small tomatoes ½ cup 3 tbsp	Mash sardine, add flour and chopped tomato. Add water, stir well; drop by tablespoons in hot fat. Fry until lightly brown.	5 min (Cooking time 10 min)	6-8 fritters (Child's portion 2 fritters)
Sweet potato and fish Cooked Sweet Potato Cooked Fish Liquid (in which potato was cooked) Margarine	4-6 tbsp 1 tbsp 3 tbsp 2 tsp	Mash potato; add flaked fish, cooking liquid and margarine and mix together	5 min	6-8 tbsp (Child's portion 6-8 tbsp)
Soup with carrot and soft dumplings Beans Water Corned Meat Cocoyam Carrots	1 cup 6 cups ¼ lb. ¼ lb. ¼ lb.	Soak meat in water (which will be thrown away). Soak beans in 6 cups water. Add meat and cook. Cook soaked beans	2 hours soaking 1 hour (preparation and	4 servings (Child's portion: 1 cup soup with beans,

Foods to use	How much	How to make	Prep. cooking time	Amount
		and meat until tender. Add scraped, diced carrots and peeled cocoyam cut in small pieces.	cooking	meats carrots and soft dump-lings.
Soft dumplings Flour Margarine Milk or Water	1 cup 1 tsp ¼ cup	Combine flour, margarine and milk/water to make dumplings and add to pot.	10 min	

IDEAS AND SUGGESTIONS FOR LEARNING ABOUT YOUNG CHILD FEEDING

What to teach	What to do	Who/What to use
Purpose: To describe how babies are introduced to new foods in addition to breast milk.		
Messages: — Breast milk is the only food baby needs for the first four months of life.	Bring in mothers who have successfully breast-fed for at least 4 months to talk about the experience.	Flip Chart "Feeding Your Baby 4-6 months and 6 months and over"
— From 4-6 months old baby needs other nourishing foods in addition to breast milk	Show how to make dif-ferent porridges and fruit juices using easily available ingredients.	Real Foods. Kitchen equipment and utensils Food Group Charts
— New foods should be fed to baby from a clean cup with a clean spoon.	Ask mothers to bring in their babies and feed them with the food pre-pared, using cup and spoon.	Real Foods Mothers and their babies.

What to teach	What to do	Who/What to use
— Feeding bottles and teats should never be used to feed baby.		
— At six months and over, baby can start eating foods cooked for the rest of the family. These foods should be mashed, strained and softened by adding gravy, margarine, butter, etc.	Demonstrate food preparation methods.	Real Foods Kitchen equipment and utensils.
— The number of meals and amount of food given to the young child are very important.	Demonstrate quantities of food to be served.	Real Foods Kitchen equipment and utensils.
— Since baby is growing very fast he needs nourishing foods often.	Ask what the mothers feed their babies each day. Discuss how they can improve their children's diets.	Real Foods Pictures of well-and malnourished children.
— Baby's meals should be prepared according to the balanced diet principle.	Talk about the preparation of balanced meals.	Cooked meals Food Group Charts
— Baby should be taken to the clinic or health centre regularly for check-ups and immunization.	Remind mothers to take their babies to clinic at the given date.	
— Children who are sick should not be starved.		
	Questions for Discussion: When should a baby be given other foods besides breast milk?	

What to teach	What to do	Who/What to use
	What are the first foods to be given to a baby besides breast milk? Should a baby be given his porridge in a feeding bottle? Can a baby eat from the family pot? At what age? Should baby's foods which are taken from the family pot be specially prepared? How can a mother tell that her baby is getting enough to eat?	

10

Malnutrition in young children

Signs of good nutrition

Growth charts

Protein — energy malnutrition

Children who are likely to become malnourished

Children needing special help

Preventing malnutrition — some messages for mothers

Anaemia in young children

Ideas and suggestions for learning about malnutrition in young children

Health
Food and Nutrition

What you should be able to do after studying this chapter

After studying this Chapter, taking part in discussions and doing the exercises and activities, you should be able to:
— identify children who are not growing well;
— show a mother/childminder how to watch a child's growth;
— know the causes of protein-energy malnutrition;
— identify children who have protein-energy malnutrition;
— show mothers/childminders how to feed children who have protein-energy malnutrition;
— know the causes of anaemia;
— identify children who have anaemia;
— show mothers/childminders how to feed children who have anaemia;
— show mothers/childminders how to feed sick children.

SIGNS OF GOOD NUTRITION

All parents want their babies to look healthy and well nourished.

A child who is healthy and getting enough of the right kinds of food is alert, vigorous and active.

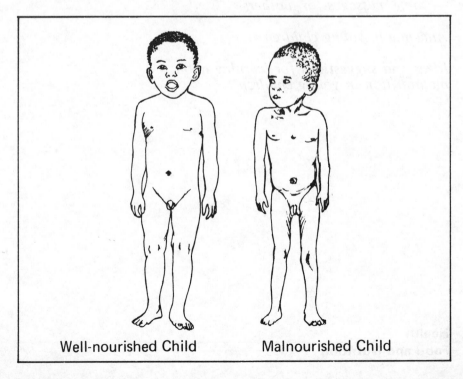

Well-nourished Child   Malnourished Child

His/her:
— Posture is good.
— Weight is in good proportion to height and age.
— Skin is clean, smooth and soft.
— Eyes are bright and clear with the inside lower eyelid and mouth bright pink.
— Tongue is pink, uncoated and moist.
— Fingernails are pink.
— Muscles are firm and well developed.
— Teeth are clean, well-formed and free from cavities.
— Breath is fresh.

Children must grow. In order to grow, they must have plenty of food. When children do not get enough food, or when they get the wrong kinds of food, they become malnourished. When a child is well-nourished he will grow well. We can tell that he is well-nourished and growing if he puts on weight.

To know if a child is putting on weight, we must weigh him regularly for the first three years of his life and record his weight on a growth chart.

GROWTH CHARTS

In most countries children under five are taken periodically to child health clinics for check-ups. At the clinic they are weighed and their weights are 'plotted' on growth charts. These measurements will tell how healthy they are and whether or not they are eating the right foods.

There are a wide variety of weight for age charts in use. Those produced by TALC have been designed from information gained from over 200 charts collected from around the world. As their kilogram lines are exactly a centimetre apart they can be used in the new low cost scales which allow direct plotting on the chart.

> **If a child's growth curve falls between the lower solid line and the dotted line the child is moderately malnourished.**
> **If the curve falls below the dotted line, the child is severely malnourished.**

If weight charts are to be successfully used then staff need to be carefully taught how to use them. For this there is a useful flannel graph available from TALC. Emphasis is always on the direction of the child growth curve. If it is going up parallel to the lines this is alright. If the curve is flattened the child may not be getting enough energy. Check the

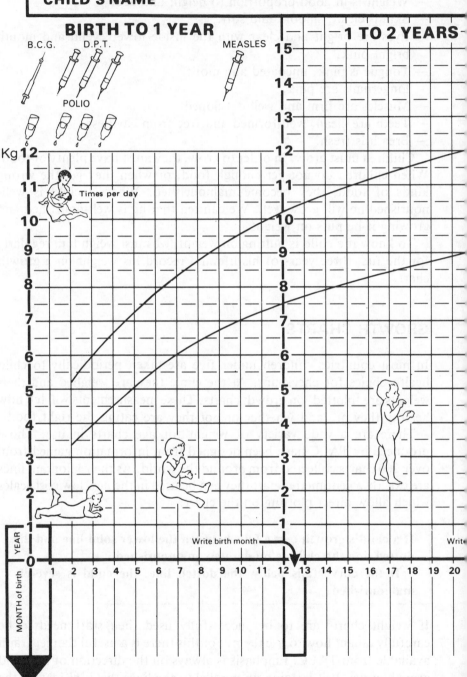

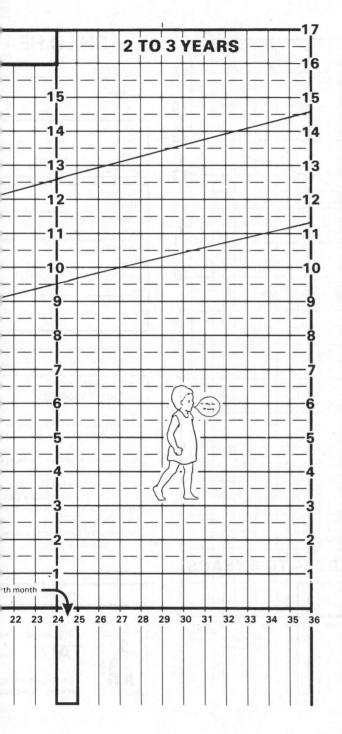

2 TO 3 YEARS

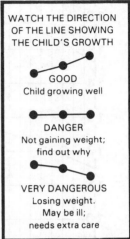

WATCH THE DIRECTION
OF THE LINE SHOWING
THE CHILD'S GROWTH

GOOD
Child growing well

DANGER
Not gaining weight;
find out why

VERY DANGEROUS
Losing weight.
May be ill;
needs extra care

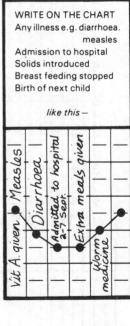

WRITE ON THE CHART
Any illness e.g. diarrhoea.
                    measles
Admission to hospital
Solids introduced
Breast feeding stopped
Birth of next child

like this —

Vit. A. given Measles Diarrhoea Admitted to hospital 2–7 Sept. Extra meals given Worm medicine

th month

22 23 24 25 26 27 28 29 30 31 32 33 34 35 36

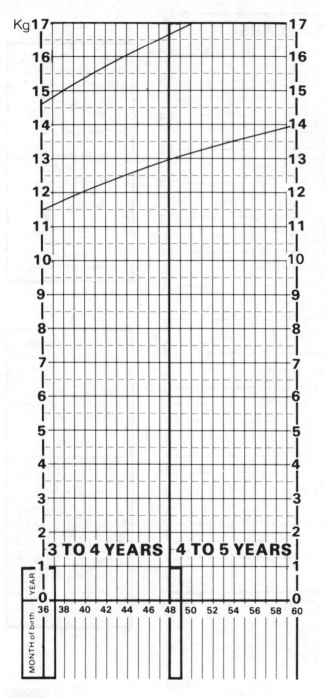

chart produced by

TALC   T
*Tr *

GROWTH CURVE Refer
UPPER LINE: 50th CENT

CHILD HEA

CLINIC 1 _____

CLINIC 2 _____

| CHILD'S NAME | |
| DATE OF BIRTH | day   month   year |

MOTHER'S NAME	
CARETAKER IF NOT THE MOTHER	
FATHER'S NAME	
WHERE DOES THE CHILD LIVI	

How many children has the mothe
Number alive _____

CARD GIVEN AND
MOTHER TAUGHT BY

*ASK THE MOTHER ABOUT THESE *
*THE CHILD EXTRA CARE (make a circ *

Was the baby **less than 2.5 kg at b**
Is this baby a **twin** _____
Is this baby **bottle fed** _____
Does the mother have **family supp**
Are any brothers or sisters **underw**
Are there any other reasons for **tak**
For example — tuberculosis or lepro

*Remember to disc *

3 TO 4 YEARS   4 TO 5 YEARS

TH CHART

_____ No _____

_____ No _____

	GIRL
	BOY

BIRTH WEIGHT	

d? _____

Number dead _____

SONS FOR GIVING *und the right answer)*	TAKE EXTRA CARE
_____ no ___	yes
_____ no ___	yes
_____ no ___	yes
_____ no ___	yes
ht _____ no ___	yes
extra care? ___ no ___	yes

or **social problems**

_____

_____

_____

s child spacing

P.O. BOX 49, ST. ALBANS, UK.
ng materials are also available

e values - **WHO recommended 1980**
BOYS LOWER LINE: 3rd CENTILE GIRLS

IMMUNISATIONS		DATE GIVEN
BCG		
POLIO	FIRST DOSE	
	SECOND DOSE	
	THIRD DOSE	
	FOURTH DOSE	
DPT Diptheria Whooping Cough Tetanus	FIRST DOSE	
	SECOND DOSE	
	THIRD DOSE	
MEASLES		
MOTHER'S TETANUS TOXOID (or one booster)	FIRST DOSE	
	SECOND DOSE	
	THIRD DOSE	

ORAL REHYDRATION
DATES

Taught			
Used			

Date of visit _____

_____

_____

_____

_____

_____

_____

_____

_____

_____

_____

_____

_____

_____

_____

_____

_____

_____

_____

_____

_____

number of meals the child is receiving. Most children need 4-5 meals a day. If the mother works could a relative give the child an extra meal? Then we need to check the energy concentration of the foods. Is the mother adding sufficient oil and fats?

In the past we used to encourage protein foods now more emphasis is placed on an adequate calorie intake by frequent meals particularly if the child has been recently unwell.

MONITORING NUTRITION AND HEALTH OF THE INDIVIDUAL CHILD

Every child should gain weight at each regular visit to the clinic. But this is not always so. Here's how to find out. Weigh the child, plot the weight on the growth chart and compare with his previous weight. If he has gained weight, his growth line or curve is going upward (/). This is good. If the child has not gained weight, his weight is more or less the same as it was the last time or two. His growth line is flat (—). This is **dangerous**. There is something wrong with the child. Find out and do something about it. If the child has lost weight and his curve is sloping down (\), it is **very dangerous**. The child needs immediate help. Do something right away to remove the causes of the loss of weight and help the child to start gaining weight again. **This is how an individual child is monitored**.

CLINIC VISITS

Ages to bring child to clinic	Dates when appointments given by the clinics					
	Schedule	√	X	Reschedule	√	X
1 month						
2 months						
3 months						
4 months						
5 months						
6 months						
9 months						
12 months						
15 months						
18 months						
21 months						
24 months						
30 months						
42 months						
54 months						

√ = Kept appointment; X = Did not keep appointment

HOME, HOSPITAL OR DOCTOR VISITS

Date	Remarks/Diagnosis	Initial	Date	Remarks/Diagnosis	Initial

SUGGESTED FEEDING SCHEDULE FOR THE FIRST YEAR OF LIFE

TYPES OF FOOD	1 MONTH	2 MONTHS	3 MONTHS	4 MONTHS	5 MONTHS	6 MONTHS	7 MONTHS	8 MONTHS	9 MONTHS	10 MONTHS	11 MONTHS	12 MONTHS
BREAST MILK												
FRUIT (PUREE OR JUICE)												
THICK PORRIDGE (WITH MILK)												
SOLT/SOFT FAMILY MEAL												

TAKE - HOME GROWTH CHART

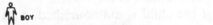 BOY

Health Centre	Regd. No.
Child's Name	Date of birth
Mother's name:	
Guardian's name (if other than mother):	
Where the child lives (Address)	

BROTHERS AND SISTERS

Year of Birth	Boy/ Girl	Remarks	Year of Birth	Boy/ Girl	Remarks

IMMUNIZATIONS

WHOOPING COUGH, TETANUS AND DIPHTHERIA		POLIOMYELITIS		When to Get
	Date Given		Date Given	
First dose				Three doses by 7 months at least 1 month apart
Second dose				
Third dose				
First booster				18 months
Second booster				3-6 years

TUBERCULOSIS (BCG) (birth or 3 months)	MEASLES (9 to 15 months)	RUBELLA (9 to 15 months)
Date Given	Date Given	Date Given

OTHERS, Type and Date

LANDMARKS OF DEVELOPMENT

	Normal Age Range
Balances head at ____ months	3-6 months
First tooth at ____ months	5-8 months
Sitting without support ____ months	5-11 months
Able to walk few steps ____ months	12-15 months
Able to speak 4-5 single words ____ months	15-21 months
Toilet trained ____ months	24-36 months

Here is a summary of how you go about monitoring the individual child at the clinic.

1. Register the child, record or update basic information.
2. Weigh the child.
3. Plot the weight on the clinic and take-home charts.
4. Measure the child's height if needed and haemoglobin (Hb) level (for anaemia) if required, and record.
5. Note the feeding pattern, major illnesses, or other factors which affect the child's nutrition.
6. Fill in all necessary information on the take-home and clinic charts.
7. Explain the growth curve to the parents.
8. Compliment the parents if the child is well-nourished and encourage them to keep it up. This is as important as letting the parents know if their child is getting malnourished. Remind them about the date of the next clinic visit.

If the child is malnourished, find out why.

(a) It may be due to illness. Refer to treatment and guide on proper feeding during illness.
(b) It may be due to feeding problems even though there is enough food.
(c) It may be due to not enough food. Provide supplementary foods if available, or refer to Social Services or other ways to obtain foods.

Follow-up with home visits or refer to one who will visit. Remind parents of date of next clinic visit. **A malnourished child needs very close follow-up**.

MONITORING THE COMMUNITY FOR HEALTH AND NUTRITION OF CHILDREN

This is done in three steps:
1. Knowing all the children in the community.
2. Following up the children in the community.
3. Preparing a monthly summary of the situation for decision-making, action and keeping track of what is happening.

Knowing and following up all the children in the community

A health centre serves all the children in the community — those who come to the clinic and those who do not come. Thus it is not enough to monitor only those children who come to the clinic.

You must know about all the children in your community.

This can be done as follows:

1. Update the list of children 0-4 years in each community. At first you may have to make door-to-door visits to prepare this list. Later you can update by keeping a list of births, deaths and those who have left the country (migrated). A volunteer in the community can make this list for you.
2. Prepare a growth chart for all children in the community. You may end up with three groups:
   (a) Those who come to the clinic.
   (b) Those who go to private doctor or other services.
   (c) Those who do not get any services.
3. File the charts alphabetically by sex, separately for each community or area.
4. Before visiting the community go through the charts and prepare a list of not only those who come to the clinic and need help, but also those who should have come to the clinic but did not. As you visit the community, persuade the defaulters to come to the clinic.
5. On your return to the clinic, discuss your findings with your supervisor and ask for assistance if needed.

Preparing a monthly summary of the situation

You need to know what is happening in your community. Is the situation improving? Is the situation getting worse? The answers lie in preparing a picture of the situation in the community periodically. This can be done as follows:

1. Every month pull out the growth charts of those who were supposed to attend clinic that month, and those who did attend. This will give you the coverage by your clinic.
2. Of those who attended clinic that month, how many have growth curves below the lower solid line? These are malnourished children for that month. Compare this figure with last month's figure. This will give you an idea if the situation has been improving or getting worse.
3. Prepare your work plan according to the needs of the communities. There are problems which you can solve without much extra assistance. List them and go after them.
4. Prepare a list of those problems which you cannot solve and inform your supervisors, suggesting the type of assistance needed.
5. If and when there is extra assistance, incorporate it in your work plan.

   These steps constitute community-level monitoring of the nutritional status of children. A Field Guide, which is available at health centres, sets out the procedures step by step.

> **Remember! To monitor the nutrition of the individual child, follow the weight gain pattern of that child compared to his or her previous weight. To monitor the community, count the children whose weight falls below the lower solid line on the growth chart and compare with figures from the previous time. Do not wait for the individual child's weight to fall below the lower solid line to provide assistance.**

PROTEIN-ENERGY MALNUTRITION (PEM)

> **Weighing a child regularly, plotting the weights on a growth chart and noting the direction of the growth curve are the most important steps in recognizing early malnutrition.**

Being underweight for age is a common form of malnutrition in young children. The underweight child could become severely malnourished. He may get infections easily. The child may not grow and develop well to be a productive adult.

The first sign of all forms of protein-energy malnutrition is growth failure. The child is thinner and shorter than normal. Growth failure can be seen most clearly on a child's growth chart. Weeks or months before a child looks like a case of malnutrition he will have stopped growing.

A community worker should be able to identify children with malnutrition at the earliest possible stage in order to cure them more effectively.

The severe forms of protein-energy malnutrition are described below. There are two main types of severe PEM:
— Marasmus
— Kwashiorkor

Some children have features of both types of PEM. These children have **marasmic kwashiorkor.**

Marasmus
Children get marasmus when they do not eat as much good food as they need.

Children with marasmus:
— have no fat (very skinny);
— are very underweight — 'all skin and bones';
— have an 'old person's' face;
— are always hungry.

Many children get marasmus between the age of 6-14 months during the weaning period.

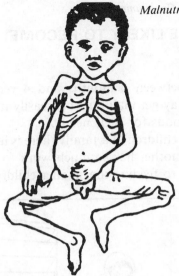

From age 4 months all babies need more food in addition to breast milk.

Kwashiorkor

Kwashiorkor may start at a later age than marasmus. Often it starts between age 18 and 48 months. It is a serious sickness especially when there are the added complications of infection. It needs urgent medical care.

Children with kwashiorkor:
— show body swelling (oedema), especially on the legs and feet and sometimes on the face,
— have soft, flabby muscles,
— have cracked, peeling skin,
— have thin, reddish hair,
— are unhappy and often peevish and may not want to eat.

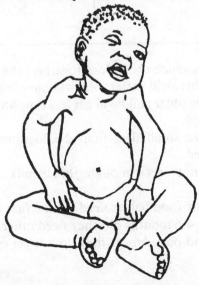

CHILDREN WHO ARE LIKELY TO BECOME MALNOURISHED

1. When children are between 6 months and 4 years old they are growing fast. They may get malnourished easily if they do not get enough of the right foods for their needs.
2. When there are many children in a family there is less food for each person. Because the mother has so much work to do she may not pay enough attention to feeding the smaller children.

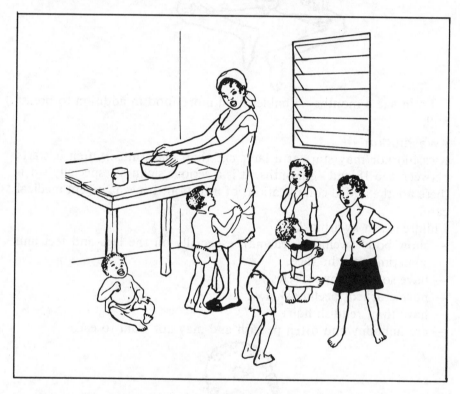

3. If a mother has pregnancies too close together, the health of both babies, and the mother, will suffer. She will have less breast milk to feed the baby and the older child will get less time and care and may become malnourished.
4. Babies who are born small (less than 2 kilograms) are likely to become malnourished.
5. Babies who do not get enough breastmilk may become malnourished.
6. Breast milk is the only food babies need for the first four months of life, but from about 4-6 months old they need other foods, such as fruits, fruit juices and porridge. If they do not get enough of these

other foods at the right time, they will not grow properly. They may become malnourished.

7. If a child catches an infection such as diarrhoea, whooping cough or measles, he is likely to become malnourished.

8. By the time a baby is 3 months old he should be about 1.5 kilograms heavier than he was when he was born. If he gains less, he may become malnourished. Stopping breastfeeding too early can cause the baby to stop growing.

9. Poor families often cannot afford to buy or grow enough food for everyone in the family. The younger children are usually the ones who do not have enough to eat and may become malnourished.

10. If a family or community does not know how to feed children properly, they often do not get enough of the right kinds of food, and are likely to become malnourished.

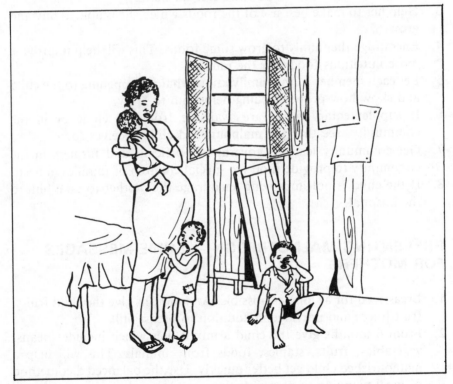

CHILDREN NEEDING SPECIAL HELP

1. Children who are likely to become malnourished (see 1-10 above).
2. Children already suffering from malnutrition.
3. Children who also have diseases like anaemia, or diarrhoea and fever very often.

4. Children who do not have very serious malnutrition but who do not improve with feeding and other help from the community worker. These children must be sent to the health centre or hospital.

The community worker can help most children who do not have very serious malnutrition. Some children need special care because they could die. Examples of these are those with serious malnutritions — very thin children with marasmus, or very swollen kwashiorkor children who won't eat.

Special help which the Community Worker can give malnourished children and their families

1. Visit these families more often than others.
2. Show the mother how the child can eat better.
3. Help her to make best use of the foods which she is able to buy and grow.
4. Encourage the family to grow some foods. This will help to provide more nutritious foods for the family.
5. Let each member of the family know what is happening to the child and show how proper feeding helps him to grow.
6. If supplementary foods are available from the clinic or in the community, see that the malnourished child receives some.
7. Get community leaders, government officials and farmers in the community to provide food for special children of families in need.
8. If the child is not improving encourage the mother to take him to the hospital.

PREVENTING MALNUTRITION — SOME MESSAGES FOR MOTHERS

1. Breastfeed for as long as possible. At 4 months give the child fruits, fruit juices and porridge in addition to breast milk.
2. From 6 months give the child a mixed diet which includes beans, vegetables, fruits, staples, foods from animals. This will help a malnourished child get better quickly. Use the balanced diet method of meal planning to plan nutritious meals.
3. Give more meals per day. This a good way of giving more food. A child with malnutrition needs six meals per day. He should get good portions of food, not just snacks.
4. Add fat to the meals. Use cooking oils, butter or margarine to add more energy to the meal and make the food better tasting so that the child eats more.

Watching a child with malnutrition get better is very encouraging to both the community worker and the child's parents. Weigh the child regularly so that the improvement is easy to see.

Talk about the results with the parents (and grandparents if necessary). This is a good way to teach the importance of good nutrition.

ANAEMIA IN YOUNG CHILDREN

Anaemia is the name given to the condition when the blood has too few red blood cells or too little of the red pigment haemoglobin. Haemoglobin carries oxygen to all parts of the body for their normal functioning. Anaemia is also referred to as having 'weak' or 'thin' blood.

How can we tell if a child has anaemia?
The best way is to have the blood checked at the clinic.

The child may be less active than normal. The child may have infections often. If you look at the inside of the lips and lower eyelids and they are a light pink or whitish instead of bright pink, the child is anaemic. A good time to look at the child's eyelids is when he is feeding at the breast. Always look at a malnourished child to check for signs of anaemia.

What are the possible causes of anaemia?
The most common cause of anaemia is a lack of foods with plenty of iron. The body cannot make enough red blood if it does not have enough iron. The child who is growing very fast need more iron to make blood. If his main food after the first 4 months is milk, which contains very little iron, he may get anaemia. If the foods rich in iron, such as leafy green vegetables and beans, are not given to a young child regularly, he may get anaemia.

A baby may start life with too small a store of iron because his mother was anaemic during pregnancy or because he was born too early.

Losing blood inside the body, such as through worms (hookworm and whipworm) may cause anaemia.

Children who may get anaemia
Children who are:
1. born early;

2. born to anaemic mothers;
3. fed too long on only milk;
4. infested with parasites such as hookworm and whipworm;
5. not eating a mixed diet which contains iron-rich foods.

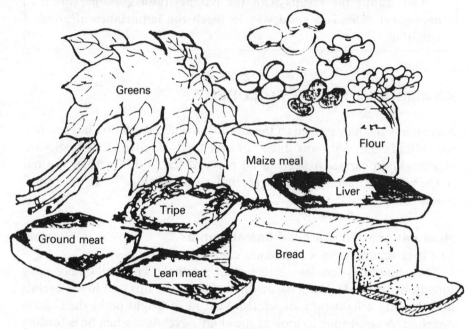

Preventing anaemia in young children

1. Pregnant women should eat different kinds of food, especially those with plenty of iron, such as dark green leafy vegetables, beans, whole grain and enriched cereals, dark brown sugar, meat and liver.
2. Pregnant women should also take iron tablets. This will build up the iron in their blood so that they can pass on a full amount to their babies before birth.
3. Babies born early (premature) need small doses of extra iron in the first 3 months of life. These will be given at the health centre.
4. After about 4-6 months, babies should have a mixed diet which contains good food sources of iron.
5. Babies should not drink tea (the common type bought in the shop) because it slows down the body's use of iron.
6. Fruits or fruit juices which taste sour, like oranges or grapefruits, help the body use the iron in foods. They should be taken with meals which contain plenty of iron.
7. Children should live in clean surroundings, use the toilet and wear shoes where possible to prevent their getting hookworm and whipworm infections.

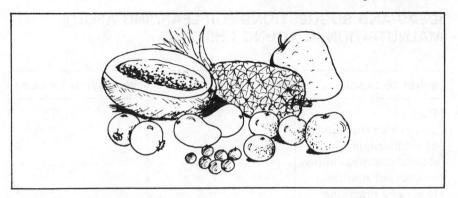

Treating a child with anaemia
— Give plenty of iron-rich foods.
— Give an iron tonic.
— Give the iron tonic after a meal so that it doesn't upset him.

> **Sickle cell anaemia is a special type of blood disease. It needs special treatment — not iron tablets.**

The child's bowel movements may be black in colour if he is taking iron. This is normal. Keep iron and other medicines out of children's reach.

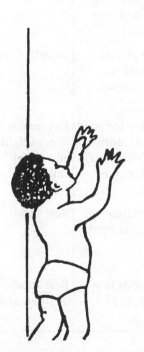

IDEAS AND SUGGESTIONS FOR LEARNING ABOUT MALNUTRITION IN YOUNG CHILDREN

What to teach	What to do	Who/What to use
Purpose: To describe the causes of malnutrition. To show that eating proper amounts of nutritious foods and practising good hygiene will help to prevent it.		
Messages: — Babies should be taken to the health clinic regularly for check-ups.	Describe the signs of good health and nutrition.	Pictures/photographs of healthy well-nourished children. Pictures of malnourished children. Real children.
— Weighing a child and plotting his weight on a growth chart, shows how well he is growing.	Show how a child is weighed. Show how a child's weight is marked on a growth chart and how to read the chart.	Scales for weighing. Growth charts.
— Poor growth leads to Protein-energy malnutrition (PEM).	Explain good growth and poor growth as shown on the growth chart.	Growth Charts
— The child who is malnourished and then eats enough good food becomes healthy.	Discuss reasons for poor growth or malnutrition. Talk about children who are likely to become malnourished.	Pictures of healthy, underweight, marasmic and kwashiorkor children.
— After illness children need to eat more food to replace what they lost when ill.	Show why children who are malnourished need more food.	Real foods.
— Anaemia is a kind of malnutrition.	Talk about foods that are good sources of iron.	Real foods/Pictures of foods rich in iron.

What to teach	What to do	Who/What to use
— Anaemia can be prevented by eating foods that are rich in iron.		
— Clean food, clean water, clean hands, clean utensils prevent sickness.	Demonstrate proper hand-washing using clean water, soap and towel. Talk about how germs are spread by dirty personal habits.	Basin with water; soap in dish; towel

11

Diarrhoea

What is diarrhoea?

How to feed the child who has diarrhoea

How to feed the child who is dehydrated

How to prevent diarrhoea

*Ideas and suggestions for learning
about diarrhoea*

**Health
Food and Nutrition**

WHAT YOU SHOULD BE ABLE TO DO
AFTER STUDYING THIS CHAPTER

After studying this chapter, taking part is discussions and doing the exercises and activities, you should be able to:
— Help mothers/childminders understand what causes diarrhoea.
— Show mothers/childminders how to feed children with diarrhoea.
— Show mothers/childminders how to prepare the Oral Rehydration Solution (ORS)
— Show mothers/childminders how to feed their children after diarrhoea
— Recognize the signs of dehydration
— Show mothers/childminders how to feed children who are dehydrated.
— Show mothers/childminders how they can prevent diarrhoea

WHAT IS DIARRHOEA?

Diarrhoea is an infectious disease. We also know this as 'running belly'. When a child has diarrhoea he passes three or more loose or watery stools in one day. The stools may also contain slime and/or blood. The most obvious sign of diarrhoea is when the stools turn from yellow to green.

> **A very young breastfed baby has many stools that may be soft or watery. This is not diarrhoea.**

What causes diarrhoea?
Diarrhoea is caused by very, very small germs. They enter through the mouth and go into the belly. Germs grow wherever it is not clean and when we practise dirty habits. Some of these are:
— touching food with dirty hands;
— drinking dirty water;
— using dirty cooking and eating utensils;
— using dirty feeding bottles and teats to feed babies;
— allowing flies, dust and dirt to get onto food;
— eating dirt and playing in dirty places.
  Diarrhoea is also caused by malnutrition. When a child is malnourished he cannot digest his food normally. Malnutrition also weakens the walls of his stomach so that it cannot absorb food well. When his food is not digested and absorbed properly he gets diarrhoea.

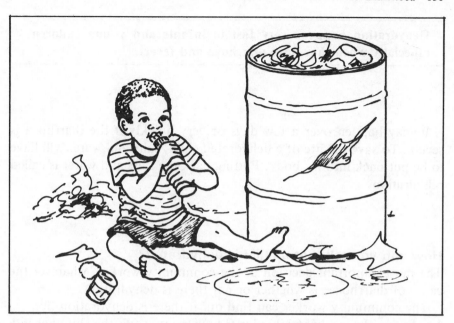

Why is diarrhoea dangerous?

Because the food is not properly absorbed, the child becomes malnourished and needs foods to make him better.

The child will also lose water and salts from his body. If he is only passing a few watery stools, he will not become dehydrated. But if he is passing many watery stools, he will become dehydrated.

Too much dehydration may cause death.

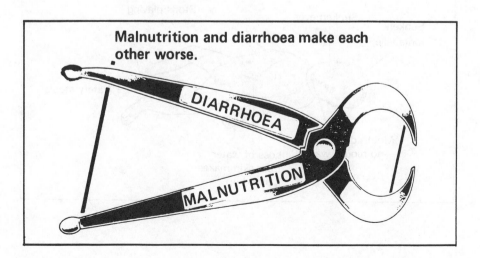

Malnutrition and diarrhoea make each other worse.

DIARRHOEA

MALNUTRITION

Dehydration happens very fast in infants and young children, especially when they have diarrhoea and fever.

It may happen over a few days or very quickly if the diarrhoea is severe. To save the life of a dehydrated child, salts and water will have to be put back into his body. Putting back the salts and water is called **rehydration**.

How can you tell that a child is dehydrated?

The most important decision of the community worker, whatever the cause of diarrhoea, is whether or not there is dehydration.

The community worker can find out if there is dehydration by:

1. Asking the mother/childminder how many stools the child has in a day or whether he feels lighter than usual.
2. Looking at the child's eyes, mouth and the colour of the urine.
3. Pinching the child's skin to see whether it will stand up.
4. Weighing the child.

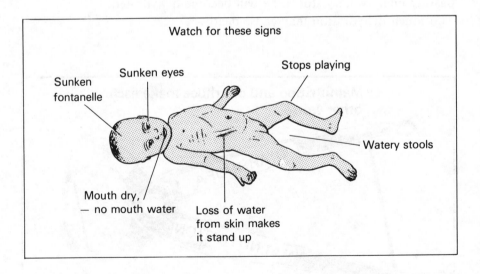

Watch for these signs

Sunken fontanelle

Sunken eyes

Stops playing

Watery stools

Mouth dry, — no mouth water

Loss of water from skin makes it stand up

Very special treatment must be given at once to the child who:
— cannot and will not drink,
— is unconscious or having fits,
— is not passing any urine,
— is passing blood in stools,
— is hot with fever,
— is malnourished.

The child with these symptoms is most likely to die if he is not taken to the Health Centre or hospital quickly.

Action	Treat child at home with plenty of liquids, such as breast milk, coconut water, clear soup or broth, clear tea, fruit juice, ORS solution. Watch for signs of dehydration.	If a child with diarrhoea has two or more of these signs, he is dehydrated. If the child who is having diarrhoea is dehydrated, he needs to be seen by the nurse or doctor for special care. If special care is not given quickly, he will die.

How to prevent dehydration

Have the child drink more fluids than usual as soon as diarrhoea starts. Coconut water, Oral Rehydration Salts (ORS) solution, thin soups or broth, lightly sweetened tea or fruit juices and milk are good fluids. If the child is breastfed, the mother should continue to breastfeed, but more often than normal (at least every 3 hours). If the child is not breastfed, he should be given full strength milk feeds every 3 hours. If full strength milk is not tolerated, give half strength milk.

CHECKING THE CHILD WHO HAS DIARRHOEA

	No dehydration	Some dehydration	Severe dehydration
1. Ask about:			
Diarrhoea	Less than 4 liquid stools per day	4 to 10 liquid stools per day	More than 10 liquid stools per day
Vomiting	None or a small amount	Some	Very frequent
Thirst	Normal	Greater than normal	Unable to drink
Urine	Normal	A small amount, dark	No urine for 6 hours
2. Look at:			
Condition	Well, alert	Unwell, sleepy or irritable	Very sleepy, unconscious, floppy or having fits
Tears	Present	Absent	Absent
Eyes	Normal	Sunken	Very dry and sunken
Mouth and tongue	Wet	Dry	Very dry
Breathing	Normal	Faster than normal	Very fast and deep
3. Feel:			
Skin	A pinch goes back quickly	A pinch goes back slowly	A pinch goes back very slowly
Pulse	Normal	Faster than normal	Very fast, weak, or you cannot feel it
Fontanelle (mole) [in infants]	Normal	Sunken	Very sunken

4. Take: Temperature	No fever	No fever	No fever
5. Weight	No weight loss	Weight loss	Weight loss
Action	Treat the child at home with plenty of fluids such as breast-milk, coconut water, clear soup or broth, clear tea, fruit juice, ORS solution and easily digested foods such as breast-milk, formulae, porridges and other mixes from the family pot. Watch for signs of dehydration.	If the child has two or more of these signs, he is dehydrated. If the child who is having diarrhoea is dehydrated, he needs to be seen by the nurse or doctor for special care. If special care is not given quickly he will die. **Take child to hospital or clinic for special care.**	

Children under 2 years old should be given ¼ to ½ cup (60-120 ml) of the ORS solution after each loose stool. Older children should get ½-1 cup (120-240 ml) ORS solution. Adults should drink as much as is tolerated. (See how to make ORS solution and how much to give below and on the next two pages.)

It is very important to feed a child foods in addition to the fluids. The child should have freshly prepared, easily digested foods. A small quantity of margarine, butter or oil should be added to the meal for extra energy. Fruit juices and bananas are especially useful as they provide a good supply of potassium. Potassium is one of the important minerals that is lost in watery stools. It must be replaced. The child should be fed 5-7 times or more often to ensure that he gets enough.

How to treat dehydration
If dehydration occurs, the child should be brought to the health centre for treatment. Here he will be given oral rehydration treatment. He gets a solution made with oral rehydration salts (ORS).

How to make ORS solution
1. Wash hands with soap and water.
2. Have ready a clean litre/quart bottle or other container and fill with clean water.
3. Cut off one corner of the packet of salts.
4. Pour the salts from the packet into the bottle.
5. Shake bottle.
6. Pour some of the mixture into a clean cup.
7. Feed the child the mixture using a clean spoon if necessary.

It is best to use cool boiled water. However, if this is not readily available, use the cleanest drinking water.

Mix fresh ORS solution each day in a clean container and keep covered. The solution must not be kept longer than 24 hours. Throw away any solution remaining from the previous day.

If the child has a large watery stool, give ½-1 cup (120-240 ml) of the solution. Give often in small amounts. If the child vomits, let him rest for about 10 minutes, then continue to give mixture, but more slowly

Do not boil the mixture after adding the salts

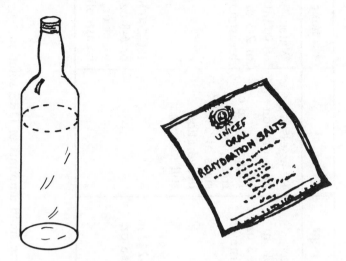

— a spoonful every 2-3 minutes. If the child drinks too quickly or if you force him to drink, he may vomit. A guide to how much ORS solution to give is given on the next page.

> **Preventing and treating dehydration with oral rehydration solution is the most important medicine for diarrhoea.**

How to mix half-strength milk
Use the same amount of water with half the amount of milk powder used to make the baby's feed when he is well.

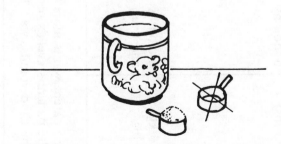

HOW MUCH ORS SOLUTION TO GIVE

Weight	Age	1st hour	2nd hour	3rd hour	4th hour
3-6 kg (6½-13 lbs)	Under 6 months	ORS 60-90 ml or 2-3 oz	ORS 60-90 ml or 2-3 oz	Water 60-90 ml or 2-3 oz or breastmilk	Water 60-90 ml or 2-3 oz or breastmilk
				Re-assess state of hydration Repeat cycle of treatment if signs of dehydration still present	
Over 6 kg or 13 lbs	6 months and over	180-240 ml or 6-8 oz	180-240 ml or 6-8 oz water or breastmilk	180-240 ml or 6-8 oz	180-240 ml or 6-8 oz water or breastmilk

- If the patent wants more ORS solution, give more.
- If the patient's eyelids become puffy, stop ORS.
- If the child vomits, wait 10 minutes and then continue slowly giving small amounts of ORS solution.

REMEMBER: While the child is getting ORS, he should be given breast milk or diluted milk feeds and other foods.

FEEDING DURING AND AFTER DIARRHOEA

It is bad to starve a child who has diarrhoea. A child who has diarrhoea may become malnourished. To grow and stay strong and resist illness better, a child must be fed enough nourishing foods.

Special attention to feeding must be given **during** and **after** diarrhoea. The child must be given nutritious foods often. **The foods recommended do not replace the need for other foods.**

What foods to give

The child less than 4 months old should continue to get milk feeds. Breastmilk is best. The child above 4-6 months of age should get foods that are very nourishing but not bulky. These foods include breastmilk, mashed fruit, juices and porridges. The child over 6 months of age should continue to be breastfed. In addition, the child should get mashed fruit, fruit juices, porridges and mixes of regular family foods such as rice, bread, potato, yam, thick soups, fish, cheese, eggs, meat, peas and soft vegetables. Oil, butter, margarine and gravy should be added to the foods to provide more energy.

Guide to Feeding

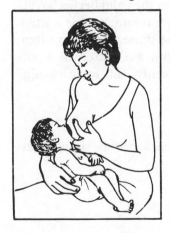 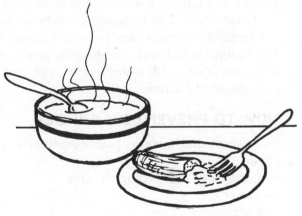

Birth to 4 months
   — breast milk
4 to 6 months old
   — thick porridge and fruit juice or mashed fruit. Breast milk.
6 months and over
   — thick porridge, fruit juice or mashed fruit, foods eaten by the rest of the family. Breast milk

About 6-12 hours after special treatment for diarrhoea, if there are no signs of dehydration, feed as usual using cup and spoon.

How to guide the mother/childminder if the same signs appear again

Should the diarrhoea get worse or signs of dehydration appear:

1. Encourage the mother (who is breastfeeding) to continue breast-feeding even more often than usual.
2. Advise the mother (who is giving formula) to stop formula feeding at once and start giving extra fluids (except milk).
3. See that the child is taken immediately to the health centre or hospital.
4. Tell the mother not to give the child foods with a lot of fibre (coarse fruits and vegetables, vegetable and fruit skins) or hot spicy foods. These will make the diarrhoea worse.
5. Advise her to give foods with plenty of energy like thick porridge with oils, fats or dark brown sugar added.
6. The child should also be given foods which contain potassium salts (pineapple, bananas, coconut water and citrus fruits and juices).
7. One extra meal each day after the diarrhoea has stopped will help the child to get stronger faster.
8. Full-strength milk should be given as soon as the child begins having fewer stools. This is usually 24-36 hours after treatment was started.

The child's bottom may get sore because he passes stools so often. The mother could wipe the bottom gently with wet cotton or a soft cloth, pat it dry with a clean, soft cloth and gently rub some vaseline over the whole bottom.

HOW TO PREVENT DIARRHOEA

To prevent diarrhoea in your community, teach people simple facts about:
— Caring for and feeding children
— Water
— Cleanliness

Caring for and feeding children

— Mothers/childminders can ensure that their children's health is carefully checked by taking them regularly to the health centre.
— One of the best ways to help prevent diarrhoea in children is to give enough food. This will help the child to gain weight each month.
— Breast milk is the BEST food for babies. It helps to prevent infections, including diarrhoea. Babies should be breastfed as often as they want.

Child's age	Breastfeeding	Milk	Other fluids	Other foods
Birth-4 months	Continue more often than usual	½ strength milk for about 6 hours	ORS/coconut water, clean water, sweetened fruit juice, sweetened tea after stool	None
4-6 months	Continue more often than usual	½ strength milk for about 6 hours	ORS/coconut water, clean water, sweetened fruit juice, sweetened tea after stool	Thick porridge, fruit juice or mashed fruit
6-12 months	Continue more often than usual	½ strength milk for about 6 hours	ORS/coconut water, clean water sweetened fruit juice, sweetened tea after stool	Thick porridge and mashed banana or mashed vegetables or thick soup

SUMMARY OF THE TREATMENT OF DIARRHOEA

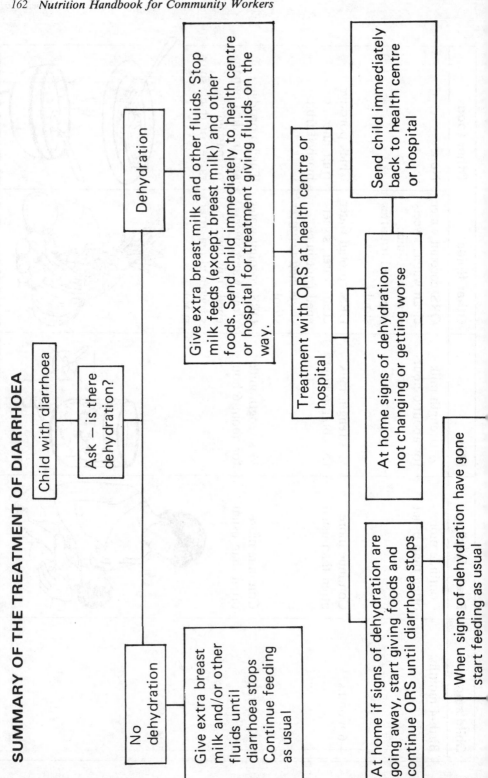

Child with diarrhoea

Ask — is there dehydration?

No dehydration

Give extra breast milk and/or other fluids until diarrhoea stops
Continue feeding as usual

Dehydration

Give extra breast milk and other fluids. Stop milk feeds (except breast milk) and other foods. Send child immediately to health centre or hospital for treatment giving fluids on the way.

Treatment with ORS at health centre or hospital

At home signs of dehydration not changing or getting worse

Send child immediately back to health centre or hospital

At home if signs of dehydration are going away, start giving foods and continue ORS until diarrhoea stops

When signs of dehydration have gone start feeding as usual

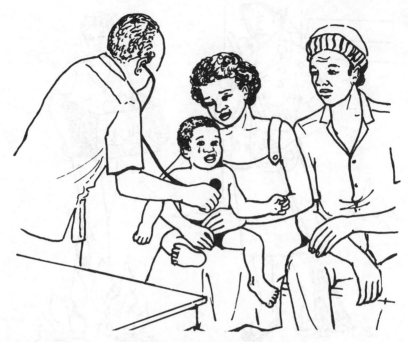

— At 4-6 months, all babies should start to have other foods besides breast milk.
— Babies should be fed from a clean cup and spoon — not a bottle. Bottles are very hard to keep clean.
— All foods should be fresh and prepared in a clean place using clean utensils.
— Cooked food should be eaten while still hot or well heated again before eating.
— Uncooked fruits and vegetables should be washed in clean water before eating.

Water
— Drinking water should be taken from the cleanest possible source and kept in a clean, covered container. If it is not certain that the water is safe, it should be boiled before drinking. Body, clothes or utensils should not be washed at the source of drinking water.
— Stools and urine should not be passed in or near the source of drinking water.

Cleanliness
Practising proper hygiene and sanitation stops germs from getting into the body:
— Rubbish should be kept in covered containers until collected burned or buried.
— The toilet and surroundings should be kept clean.

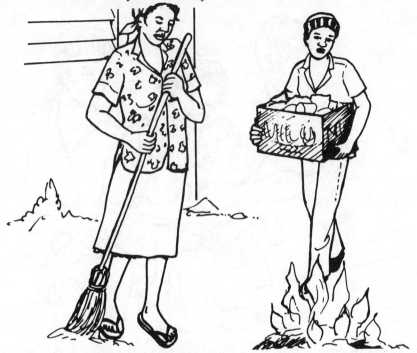

— Hands should always be washed after passing stools and before preparing food, eating, or feeding children.

Children should also learn when, why and how to wash their hands.

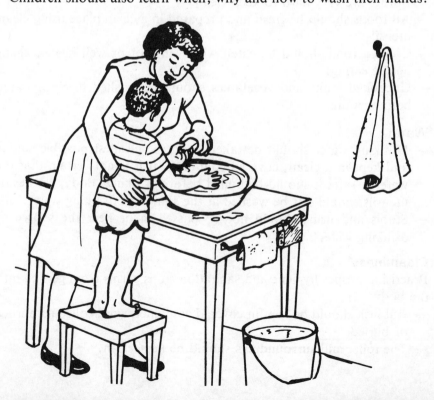

— Stools and urine should be passed in a latrine or toilet situated some distance from the source of drinking water. Stools passed by children in or near the house should be cleaned up immediately.
— Food should be kept covered to prevent contamination from flies and dust.

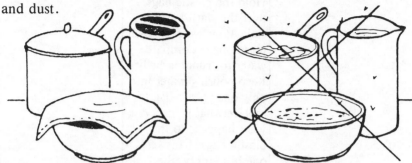

IDEAS AND SUGGESTIONS FOR LEARNING ABOUT DIARRHOEA

What to teach	What to do	Who/What to use
Purpose: To teach mothers how to control, treat and prevent diarrhoea		
Messages: — Diarrhoea is caused by germs which come from dirty hands, food, water, surroundings, cooking and feeding dishes and bottlefeeding.	Discuss the causes of diarrhoea. Show how a dirty teat and feeding bottle can spread germs. Talk about how germs are spread.	Real dirty feeding bottle and teat. Picture of dirty surroundings.
— Diarrhoea can cause dehydration due to loss of salts and water from the body.	Show poster of dehydrated child with arrows pointing to signs. Cover words with small pieces of paper and let mothers tell what the signs of dehydration are.	
— Giving fluids is the first treatment for the child with diarrhoea.	Do an experiment to show the importance of giving fluids: Make ready — 2 empty plastic bags, each with a hole in the bottom,	Empty plastic bags with holes Water in container, wash basin or sink and plastic bags

What to teach	What to do	Who/What to use
	water in a container, and wash basin or sink. Hold the plastic bags over the wash basin or sink. Pour water in each plastic bag. Compare water to 'running belly'. Keep pouring water into only one plastic bag to replace what is lost. Ask what happens to the plastic bags. (Answer: one bag empty, the other full). Compare the empty bag to the child who is not given any or enough fluid to drink. Remember: no basin is needed if the experiment is done outside. Practise this experiment first to get it right. Ask the group to think of other examples of dehydration. Give some examples:	
	— Two plants or cut flowers, one of which is put in water. The other, which is not put in water dries up, shrivels and dies.	Flowers — fresh and faded
	— An orange with a hole in end, or both ends to represent the child with diarrhoea. As you squeeze out the juice, the orange will become thinner and more wrinkled and finally, almost dry and shrivelled.	Orange

What to teach	What to do	Who/What to use
— The fluids to give during diarrhoea are breast milk, coconut water, mint tea, clear soup or broth and fruit juice.	Talk about the kinds of fluids commonly used that can be given to the child with diarrhoea.	Cup and spoon Coconut water, fruit juices, clear soup/ broth, clear tea.
— When the child with diarrhoea is not dehydrated, give fluids and food and watch for signs of dehydration.	Show how to give fluids with cup and spoon	Cup and spoon Coconut water, fruit juices, clear soup/ broth, clear tea.
— If the child with diarrhoea is getting dehydrated, give fluids and rush him to the nearest clinic or doctor.		Cup and spoon Coconut water, fruit juices, clear soup/ broth, clear tea.
— ORS is given when the child has diarrhoea.	Show mothers how to make up oral rehy-dration mixture.	Packet of ORS litre bottle Clean water Cup and spoon
— ORS can save the life of a child who is dehydrated.	Demonstrate how a mother should feed ORS to a child.	Packet of ORS litre bottle Clean water Cup and spoon Young child and mother
— The child with diarrhoea should be given food. When he is better he needs plenty of nourishing food to make up for what he has lost.	Plan nourishing meals, using the balanced diet principle.	Real Foods Food Group Chart Samples of Meals
— Diarrhoa can be pre-vented by: — proper child feeding — clean water — proper hygiene and sanitation	Discuss proper child feeding and sanitation.	Pictures of clean surroundings.

12

Feeding other groups

Nutritional needs of other groups

Schoolchildren

Teenagers

Elderly people

Ideas and suggestions for learning about feeding Other groups

**Health
Food and Nutrition**

WHAT YOU SHOULD BE ABLE TO DO
AFTER STUDYING THIS CHAPTER

After studying this chapter you should be able to:
— show mothers/childminders how to plan and serve school-age and teenage children nutritious meals;
— help parents/childminders understand how important it is to have a good breakfast;
— identify those teenagers who need special nutritional help and refer them to the health centre;
— understand the problems of the elderly and how these affect their nutrition;
— show the elderly how to plan and prepare nourishing meals.

NUTRITIONAL NEEDS OF OTHER GROUPS

Each group in the community has its own special needs for nourishing foods. It is important to recognize these special needs and to feed each group properly. Three of these groups are school children, teenagers and elderly people.

SCHOOL CHILDREN

When children reach school age, they are still growing, although not as fast as their younger brother and sisters. They are usually very active

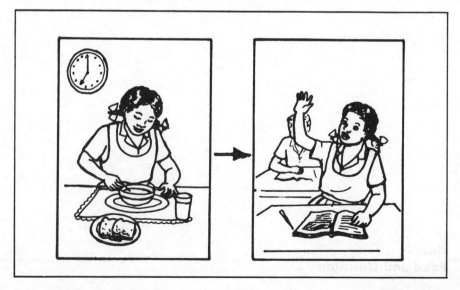

and use up plenty of energy every day. If they do not eat properly, they will not be healthy and will not grow and develop as they should. School children who don't get enough food, or enough of the right kinds of food cannot pay attention in school. Hungry children get bored easily and do not do their lessons well. Their school attendance may also be bad as they may have neither the energy nor interest to want to go to school. They may be sickly. They may have iron-deficiency anaemia.

Planning meals for children

School children need mixtures of foods from the six food groups (see page 5-6). Every day eating at least three meals containing enough foods from the food groups will help children to develop properly, stay healthy and learn well.

Since school children can easily get anaemia, parents and guardians should make sure that children of this age get foods that have plenty of iron (see page 10-14).

To help the children enjoy their meals, parents should make them appetizing. Food that is crisp, in small pieces, easy to handle and with a good blend of colours will entice children to eat.

Breakfast

A good breastfast is very important for school children. If a school child does not have breakfast before leaving home, he will not be able to pay attention during class. He may even faint.

Good breakfasts are:

Fruit + porridge + bread + butter or margarine

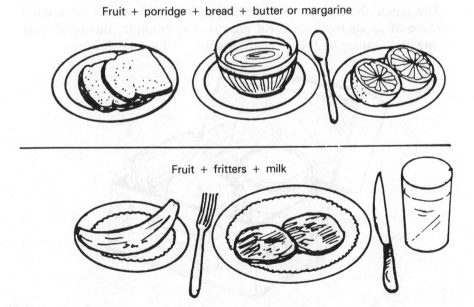

Fruit + fritters + milk

Fruit + yam or potato, fish and spinach + cocoa

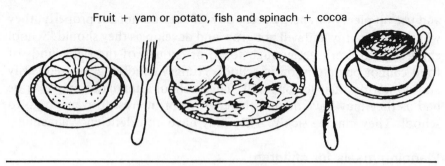

Fruit + plantain + mackerel

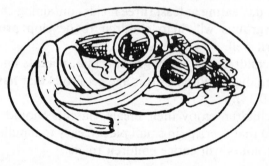

A drink of hot 'tea' alone does not provide enough nourishment.

Lunch

School children should carry a packed lunch to school or eat the school lunch. There should be enough food provided to make the child satisfied.

The lunch should also be appetizing. It should consist of a good mixture of foods from different groups. For example, flavoured milk + bread + butter with egg + groundnuts + banana + orange.

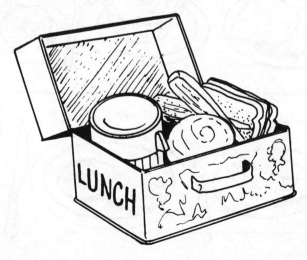

Those parents who prefer to give their children 'lunch money' should tell them what to buy with it. A soft drink, sweets, chips do not make a nourishing lunch. It is often cheaper to provide a packed lunch than to allow the children to choose from the 'goodies' available for sale outside the school.

If school children lose interest in carrying lunches to school, the school lunch might be a welcome change. They may eat the school lunch quite happily because they are eating with their friends.

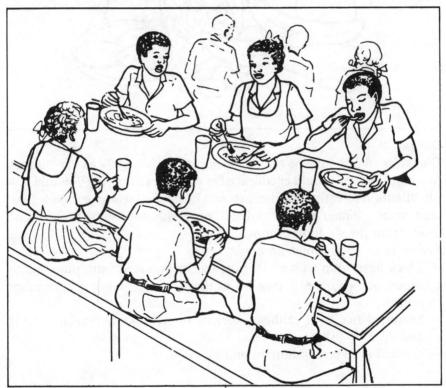

Mothers who work away from home should provide proper foods for their school-age children to eat when they come home from school. Foods like bread and groundnut paste, biscuits, milk, lemonade, fruit and fritters are nourishing. They will also encourage good eating habits.

Snacks

A banana or other fruit, a little packet of groundnuts and a few sweet biscuits can be slipped into the lunch bag along with the food provided for the mid-day meal. Children like snacks and these are more nourishing and cheaper than the 'energy only' snack foods like popsicles, soft drinks and sweets. Other good snacks are 'patties' (meat pie), sausage, milk, fruit and fritters.

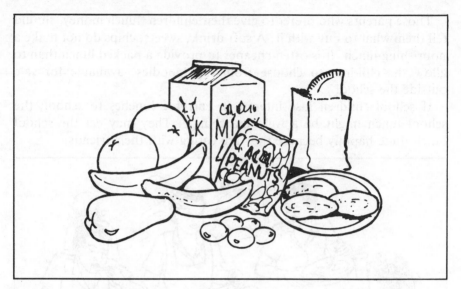

Dinner

Dinner or supper may be the one meal which the child can eat without rushing. Mothers should encourage the children to eat. They should pay full attention to eating, so there should be no distractions around. Like other meals, dinner should be based on good, nourishing mixtures of foods from the six food groups.

Examples of good dinners are:

— Thick bean soup with maize porridge or pounded yam, pumpkin (a spoon or two of milk powder in the porridge makes it even more nutritious).

— Seasoned rice with cabbage, carrots or pumpkin, spinach), beans and meat or fish.

— Canned mackerel, pumpkin and plantain.

TEENAGERS

Poor eating habits of teenagers

Teenagers often try to follow their own or their friends' eating habits. They may skip meals, eat snacks instead of 'sit-down' meals or follow 'fad' diets. Some teenage girls, who want to look very slim may go on weight reducing 'crash' diets. These practices may be bad for their health. They may become undernourished and even seriously ill if they do not eat proper, nourishing food.

Good meals and eating habits for teenagers

The teenager should have three regular meals from a variety of foods.

Use the six food groups as a guide to selecting these foods. This is the only sure way they can get all the necessary nourishment each day. Good mixtures of foods should be eaten at breakfast, lunch and dinner.

Breakfast

This could be bread and egg accompanied by porridge or milk and fruit. A good breakfast will help the teenager to do well at lessons and sports at school.

Snacks

Nourishing snacks are: fruits, fruit juices, biscuits, milk, peanuts, patties (meat pies) and fritters. These snacks should be eaten between, not instead of, regular meals.

Lunch

If the teenager is in school, a good lunch should be provided every day. It should include a good mixture of foods following the balanced diet principle. A packed lunch is cheaper and more nourishing than the snack foods sold at school. A packed lunch for a teenage girl may be one or two sandwiches and fruit or juice. For boys there may be need for three to four sandwiches.

The teenager can also eat the school lunch. It is not expensive and often nourishing. A good cooked lunch could consist of rice, fish and spinach or beans, cabbage and maize meal porridge or yam, pumpkin and meat.

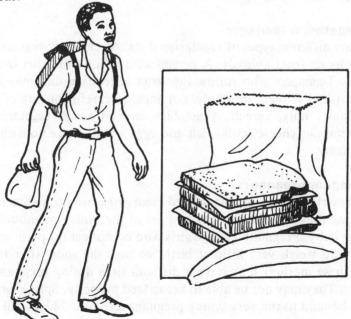

Dinner
Like other meals dinner should be based on good nourishing mixtures of foods from the food groups. The cooked lunches mentioned above can also used for dinners. Special care should be taken to include foods with plenty of iron.

Why iron is important
Teenagers should eat many different kinds of nutritious foods every day. They should pay special attention to foods with plenty of iron. Foods with plenty of iron are meats, especially liver; beans, spinach and other dark green leafy vegetables; dark brown sugar and molasses. Iron is also found in enriched breads and wheat flour. To help the body use iron well teenagers should eat fruits or drink juices with meals. Acid fruits like oranges, cherries and guavas are especially good for this purpose.

> **Iron is especially important for teenage girls who are menstruating.**

When there is not enough iron in the diet, or when the body cannot use the iron in the diet well, a teenage girl may get anaemic. Teenage boys also lose iron when they are active in sports and sweat a lot. Some teenagers who are on vegetarian diets may be anaemic because they lack iron as well as other nourishing substances.

Teenagers needing special attention

The vegetarian teenager
There are different types of vegetarian diets. A very strict vegetarian diet has no foods from animals. A person who follows this diet is called a 'vegan'. Teenagers who follow the strict vegetarian diet may become malnourished if their meals do not include careful blends of beans, groundnuts, nuts, cereals, vegetables and fruits. A vegetarian diet which contains cheese, milk, fish and eggs will be more nourishing for the teenager.

The pregnant teenager
Teenage girls who get pregnant need plenty of extra nourishment. This is because they are still growing and are at the same time nourishing a growing baby. Pregnant teenage girls who do not eat properly will have babies who weigh very little at birth, or may die soon after they are born. These mothers may have a difficult time during pregnancy and delivery. They may not be able to breastfeed properly. Special attention should be paid to the very young pregnant teenager. She is still a child

herself and at the same time has a child growing inside her who needs nourishment to develop properly. She should get plenty nourishing foods for herself and her growing baby.

The teenager with a disease related to nutrition
Teenagers with diabetes, hypertension or heart disease in their family must watch their diets carefully. Those who are suffering from these diseases should follow their special diet. Snack foods and foods from restaurants should be nourishing and eaten in small portions. Foods which are highly salted, (e.g. crisps) or high in sugar and fat (chocolates, 'french fries') should be avoided.

ELDERLY PEOPLE

When people get older they still have special needs for nourishing food. Since they are less active and use less energy, they do not need as many calories as younger people.

To cut down on calories, they should use less margarine, cooking oil, other fats, sugars, sweets and starchy foods.

Food for the elderly has to be carefully chosen and properly prepared. Make sure meals are balanced.

How to deal with problems which may affect nutrition in the elderly

Loss of teeth
— Cut food into small pieces or crush.
— Add gravy or other liquid to food to make chewing easier.
  Be sure to give nourishing foods which need little chewing and are easy to digest, e.g. thick soup, porridge and milk drinks.

Loss of appetite
— Prepare colourful and tasty meals according to the balanced diet principle.
— Serve small nourishing meals often.
— Serve meals in pleasant surroundings and allow enough time for eating slowly.

Poor digestion and constipation
— Serve fresh fruits and vegetables which do not cause indigestion.
— Serve cooked vegetables and stewed fruits if fresh ones cause indigestion.

— Include staples such as yams, plantain and maize meal in the diet.

Lack of money
— Buy low-cost, locally produced foods.
— Keep a home garden.

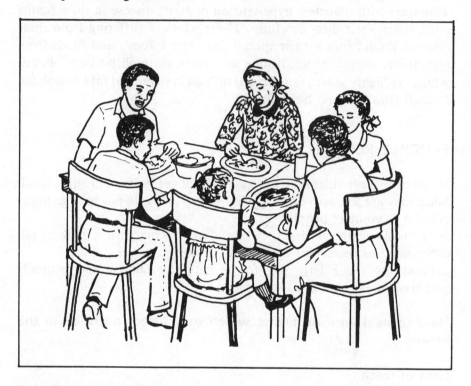

Loneliness
— Family and friends should spend time with the elderly, especially at meal times. This will encourage them to eat well and regularly.
— Help them feel a part of family and community life by giving them a part to play. For example, they could help to care for young children in the family, if they are able. They could look after a home garden and animals. This will give them useful exercise and make them feel they are making a contribution to the family. Being involved in what is going on is the best tonic available.

The older person with a disease related to nutrition
If the older person has or develops a disease or condition that requires special foods, get help from a doctor, dietitian or nutritionist. The patient must understand and follow the dietary advice. This is especially important for older people with diabetes, high blood pressure, overweight and heart disease.

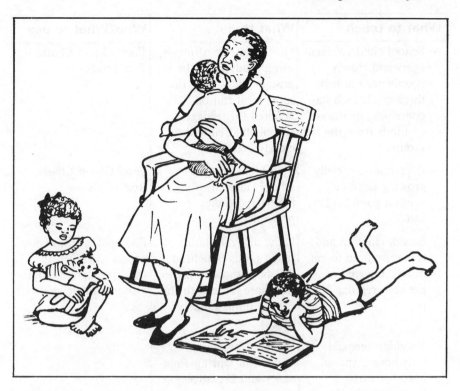

IDEAS AND SUGGESTIONS FOR LEARNING ABOUT FEEDING OTHER GROUPS

What to teach	What to do	Who/What to use
Purpose: To show that school children, teenagers and elderly people all need good nutrition and that they should be given special attention.		
Messages: — School children who do not get enough food or enough of the right kinds of food cannot do well in school.	Explain how good health and nutrition make school children attend school regularly, pay attention in class and be bright.	Samples of nourishing foods for school children

What to teach	What to do	Who/What to use
— School children, teen-agers and elderly people need at least three meals each day containing mixtures of foods from the six groups.	Give examples of meals using foods from the six groups. Show how the same meal can be adapted for teenagers, school children and elderly people.	Food Group Charts, Real foods
— Everyone, especially growing children, needs a good break-fast.	Plan breakfasts for school children, using the balanced diet principle.	Food Group Charts, Real foods
— School children and teenagers need to eat nourishing snacks between regular meals.	Show different kinds of snack foods bought at the shop, showing prices. Compare these with the cost of home-made snacks.	Food pages from news-papers. Samples of snacks bought. Samples of home-made snacks.
— Pregnant teenage girls have a special need for extra nourishing food and iron.	Review Chapter on 'Nutrition During Preg-nancy and Breastfeeding'	
— Elderly people have special problems which may affect their nutrition.	Discuss loss of teeth, loneliness, poor living conditions and other health, social and economic problems of elderly people and how they can be solved.	Social worker; nutri-tionist; elderly person who is managing his /her nutrition well.

13

Obesity

How to tell if a person is to fat (obese)

Obesity and health

Weight control

Sample menus

Some facts about exercise and weight control

Ideas and suggestions for learning about obesity and weight control

Health
Food and Nutrition

WHAT YOU SHOULD BE ABLE TO DO AFTER STUDYING THIS CHAPTER

After studying this chapter you should be able to:
— Recognize that obesity is a health problem;
— Determine how obese a person is;
— Control your weight;
— Guide people in controlling their weight.

HOW TO TELL IF A PERSON IS TOO FAT (OBESE)

Many people are too fat. When people are much too fat we say they are obese. There are many ways to tell that a person is obese. The most highly recommended way is to find the **Body Mass Index (BMI)**. To do this, divide a person's weight by his or her height in metres squared, i.e. weight in kg/height in metres². You can weigh in pounds and convert to kilograms by dividing by 2.2. You can also measure height in feet and inches and convert to metres by dividing inches by 39. (See units of Metric Measurement Annex 2.) Therefore, if a person weighs 160 pounds and is 5 feet 2 inches tall you would calculate the BMI as follows:

$$\text{Weight in kilograms} = 160 \div 2.2 = 73$$
$$\text{Height in metres} = (5 \text{ feet} \times 12 + 2) \ 62 \text{ inches} \div 39 = 1.55$$
$$\text{BMI} = \frac{\text{weight (kilos)}}{\text{height}^2 \text{ (metres)}} = 73 \div (1.55 \times 1.55) = 30$$

If the BMI is 20-24.9 that person has the right weight for height or desirable weight. If the BMI is 25-29.9 the person is classified as being in grade I obesity. If 30-40, grade II and if over 40 grade III or extremely fat.

If you have a problem doing the calculations, follow the directions and read off the BMI on the Nomogram on the next page.

Why do people become obese?

People become obese because they eat more than they need or can use and/or spend less energy than they should. Usually bottle-fed babies tend to be obese. Adults, especially those who do not do hard physical work or are not very active, are likely to become obese. They may be taking in the same amount of food energy as when they were younger, but are not active enough to get rid of some of the energy taken in as food. The energy not used up is stored as fat. Some persons tend to over-eat or to eat all the time. They may be worried, depressed, or have other

Nomogram for calculating body mass index*

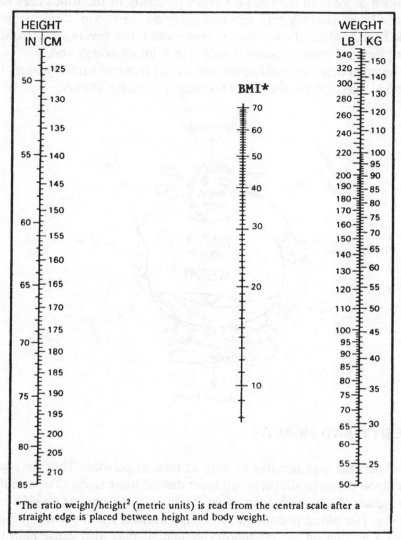

HEIGHT IN CM	BMI*	WEIGHT LB KG

*The ratio weight/height^2 (metric units) is read from the central scale after a straight edge is placed between height and body weight.

Adapted from J. Amer. Diet. Assen., 85:1117-1121, 1985.

Directions

1. Locate the person's height on the left column. Numbers in this column **increase** going down the scale.
2. Locate the person's weight on the right column. Numbers in this column **decrease** going down the scale.
3. Lay a ruler or straight edge so that it touches these two points — height and weight.
4. Note where the straight edge crosses the middle line between these two columns. This is the person's W/H^2 value or BMI.

problems, so 'make up' for these conditions by over-eating. Some people eat much more than they need. Others fry many of the foods they eat or use a lot of cooking fats, oils and gravy on their food. Some people drink a lot of alcoholic beverages, sweet and other beverages. Alcohol gives plenty of energy. Sweet foods give a lot of energy too.

In some people the breakdown and use of fats and carbohydrates in the body may not be normal. This may also cause obesity.

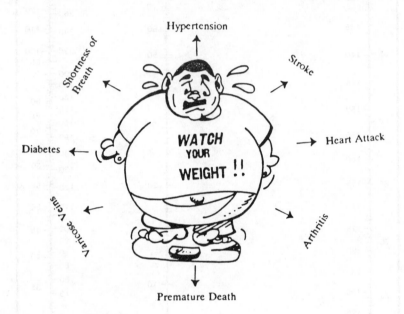

OBESITY AND HEALTH

Obese persons may not live as long as normal persons. They may get high blood pressure, diabetes and heart disease more easily than persons who are not obese. A pregnant woman who is obese may have a difficult delivery. Her blood pressure may be high because she is obese. Obesity places a burden on the circulatory system. It may also cause pain by putting pressure on the joints (in persons with arthritis). It is a risk to perform surgery on obese persons. Obese persons are likely to develop varicose veins, gout and hernias. Extra fat in and around the chest interferes with breathing and the functioning of the heart.

Obese persons may also suffer socially, mentally and financially. They may not get certain jobs. They may not be able to participate in some types of sports. The fat child may be teased or mocked by his peers and left out of some school activities. In some cases obese persons pay higher premiums for life insurance. Additional health risks arise when persons go on 'crash' diets to lose weight.

Obesity is an unnecessary, severe, physical and social handicap. Unnecessary, because it can be prevented and corrected to reduce its ill-effects. Also, it is the underlying cause of many other serious and often fatal health conditions such as diabetes, high blood pressure and heart attack.

WEIGHT CONTROL

The only way to control weight is to eat less and exercise. In other words put out more energy and take in less energy. If you take in more energy than you put out, you gain weight. If you put out more than you take in you lose weight.

Body weight is made up of many different substances. Three of these are important in understanding weight control. These are body water, protein and fat stores. Fat stores rather than body water and protein should be reduced. A person may lose as much as 5 lbs (2 kg) a day, but this weight will be water weight which may be replaced as quickly as it was lost by drinking water. If the person starves not only will body fat be lost, but muscle (protein) and water will also be lost.

If the person tries to lose weight by dieting alone, both fat and muscle (protein) will be lost. Protein will be lost even if larger portions of meat or other protein-rich food are eaten. In addition, of those who reduce weight through diet, 20% alone will keep the weight off on a long term basis. The others will go back to their original weight very quickly. When weight is lost by exercise alone, or by a combination of diet and exercise, usually fat is lost and the amount of muscle in the body is increased. The best way to reduce is to have a low calorie diet along with regular exercise.

To keep weight off permanently a person may also need to change some old habits. Dieting, exercising and changing some old habits are ways of managing obesity. Here is a guide to losing weight and keeping it off.

Dieting
Develop a healthy eating plan. Rather than going on a diet a person should develop a healthy eating plan which she is willing to follow for life. 'Going on a diet' means often selecting one of the many 'fad' diets, so popular nowadays, which the person will not want to stay on forever.

A healthy eating plan involves:

— Following a diet lower in energy or calories than the usual diet, but having all the necessary nourishing substances for good health. To get less energy from meals:

— Have smaller amounts of those foods which are high in energy such as staples (cereals, rice, bread, macaroni, dumplings, ground provisions); fats and oils; food from animals (meat, milk, cheese); sugars and sweets (rich pastry, most bottled beverages, canned or packaged juices/drinks) and alcoholic beverages (beer, stout, wine, rum and other strong liquor).

— Use skimmed milk and low fat cheese.

— Use lean meats (remove the skin from chicken).

— Boil, bake or broil foods instead of frying. Use very little, if any oil in cooking. (Remember, the foods from animals contain oil.)

— Have more vegetables.

— Use unrefined staples such as ground provisions, corn and whole wheat bread which contain fibre. Starchy foods are good sources of fibre, so should be included in the diet.

— Eat regularly. Frequent small meals will prevent a person from getting too hungry. Hunger will tempt anyone to eat foods not allowed on the plan or to overeat.

— Limit snacks to low-calorie ones such as lettuce, tomatoes, cucumbers and beverages sweetened with artificial sweeteners.

— Eat only small portions of energy-rich foods; moderate amounts of protein-rich foods (lean meat, fish, chicken, skimmed milk, peas and beans), and large amounts of fruit and vegetables, especially those with few calories (energy).

— Eat to maintain desirable weight. Once the right weight for height (desirable weight) is reached the person must eat to keep at that weight. More starchy food may be needed and about the same amount of the protein-rich foods, fruit and vegetables. Peas and beans will provide some energy and protein.

How to check on the new eating plan

— Keep a record of what is eaten for a week. That will help decide what else needs to be done in terms of cutting down or not eating some foods or eating more of others. If the plan was to have about 1,200 or 1,500 calories per day, the foods could be as shown in the sample menus on the next page.

— Weigh once per week or two, at the same time of day on the same scale. (Don't expect to lose weight all the time or as fast as at first.) A lot of water is lost in the first week on this special eating plan, but it will not happen again.

SAMPLE MENUS

1,200 Calories*

Morning: Sardine or Pilchard Salad made with:
          1 oz sardine or pilchard
          1 tsp oil + vinegar
          2 tbsp chopped tomato
          ½ tsp chopped onion
          2 small slices bread
          1 cup Coffee or Tea with:
          ½ cup Milk and artificial sweetener

Mid-morning Snack: 1 Orange

Noon Meal: Cheese Sandwich made with:
          1 oz cheese
          2 slices bread
          2 lettuce leaves
          ½ Ripe Banana
          1 cup Lemonade (artificial sweetener)

Mid-afternoon Snack: 1 small packet Peanuts

Evening Meal: 1 cup Broth (clear, thin soup)
        Stewed Chicken and Beans made with:
          2 ozs chicken (skinned)
          ⅓ cup cooked beans
          1 tsp oil
          ½ cup Rice
          1-1½ cups steamed Cabbage or Spinach
          and Pumpkin
          1 cup Cherry Juice (artificial sweetener)

Bedtime Snack: ½ cup Milk
          5 small Crackers

See amounts which make a serving — Annex 5.

1,500 Calories*

Morning: ½ Grapefruit
          1 Egg scrambled in ½ tsp Fat
          2 slices Bread
          ½ tsp Butter

Tea or Coffee with:
½ cup Milk
(sugar substitute if desired)

Noon:
3 ozs steamed Fish with Onion, Tomato,
Sweet Pepper + ½ tsp margarine
½ cup Rice & Peas
1 small boiled Green Banana (Plantain)
2 slices steamed Pumpkin
1 glass Guava Juice

Evening:
1 cup Vegetable Soup
1 stewed Chicken Leg
½ tablespoon Gravy
2 slices boiled Plantain
½ cup mashed Yam
sliced Cucumber with vinegar and pepper
1 small slice Pawpaw
1 glass Limeade
or
Cup of Tea with:
artificial sweetener, if desired

Bedtime Snack:
5 small Cream Crackers
1 small packet Peanuts
or
2 tablespoons Peanut Butter
½ cup Milk

See amounts which make a serving — Annex 5.

After about 20-30 lbs (9-14 kgs) are lost, the person's weight may stay the same. This is a good sign. If more weight is to be lost it is necessary to cut back energy-rich foods even more.

Changing bad, old habits to lose weight
It is important to take personal responsibility for losing weight. Apart from the eating and exercise plans, a person will need to replace some bad, old habits with new, good ones. For example:
— Stay away from situations which encourage eating.
— Buy only the foods on the eating plan.
— Shop when not hungry.
— Get rid of foods which should be avoided or keep them out of sight.

— Identify problems in eating and correct them. For example, food portions may be too large. A large portion of meat carries a lot of fat. Fat is very high in energy. You may be eating too fast so try to eat slowly — chew well and converse to interrupt eating.

Also try to:

— Begin a meal with a soup or a vegetable salad. This will help to make you feel full before eating too much energy-rich food.
— Have more soups or salads for main meals. A large portion of most soups is water, and salads with lots of vegetables and no oily or creamy dressings are low in calories.
— Omit sugar in tea, coffee and other beverages. Use an artificial sweetener instead.
— Use smaller plates and dishes to make smaller portions look more filling and appetizing.

Exercise

The less active a person is throughout life the fatter he or she gets. Exercise plays an important part in weight control. Why?

Exercise helps burn calories to lose body fat. It increases protein store or muscles and the rate at which the body uses energy (metabolism). It also helps to maintain the strength of muscles and flexibility of the body. Exercise prevents flabbiness as weight is lost.

Regular, vigorous exercise (aerobics) help weight loss even if the person does not diet. They also make the person lose fat stores and build muscles. The amount of weight lost may appear small, but it adds up. Exercising properly to lose weight depends on:

— the type of exercise
— how often the exercise is done (frequency)
— how vigorous the exercise is done (intensity)
— how long the exercise is done each time (duration)

Types of exercise

The best exercises are those in which the large muscles in the body are used and plenty of calories are burnt. Examples of such exercises are walking, running, rope skipping, cycling, swimming or even dancing. These rhythmic forms of exercise burn a lot of calories, reduce body fat, help keep blood pressure normal and promote fitness of the heart and blood vessels (cardiovascular system). No one type of exercise is necessarily better than the other. Each is equally effective in reducing weight, provided the frequency, intensity and duration are similar.

How often to exercise

How often the exercise is done is the key. A person should exercise regularly — at least 3-4 days per week. Less than 3 days of exercise does not help reduce body weight. If exercise is done 5-6 days per week the person will lose even more weight.

How vigorously to exercise

To lose weight or reduce fat a person should do moderate to vigorous exercises, such as running, swimming or cycling for at least 20-30 minutes each time. At each session a minimum of 300 calories should be burnt. If fewer calories are burnt little or no weight will be lost.

How long to exercise

How well exercise helps a person to lose weight depends on how long the particular exercise is done. A very fat person who starts a light exrcise such as slow walking can lose weight if the exercise is simply done for longer and longer periods of time. Of course, a very fat person puts out much more energy to perform the same task than someone of normal weight.

SOME FACTS ABOUT EXERCISE AND WEIGHT CONTROL

1. Exercise can be harmful depending on a person's state of health. A person must see a doctor before starting an exercise programme.
2. A person should not attempt to lose more than 2 lbs (1 kg) a week without a doctor's supervision.
3. An exercise programme is something a person should do for a life time. So the exercises must be enjoyable and fit into the particular lifestyle.
4. Normally, weight may go up and down by about 5 lbs (2 kgs) in a day, so a person should weigh once a week at the same time.
5. Regular exercise as described above does not increase appetite. The athlete who practises hard and for long hours does need to eat more, however.
6. Different kinds of exercises produce different results. The ones recommended here are for reducing weight. Those that are intended for muscle building and sports are different.
7. An exercise programme should be started slowly and built up to the level needed. Each exercise session should start with a warming-up for about 5 minutes and end by cooling-down for about 5 minutes. Warming-up and cooling-down are important parts of healthy exercise.
8. A person should not expect to lose weight in the early days of the exercise programme. It will be at least 2 months on an exercise

programme before one can begin to observe appreciable loss of weight.

9. A person should not try to drink too little water when beginning an exercise programme. Drinking too little water could lead to dehydration as water is lost in sweat and exhaled air.

10. Exercises done on machines, vibrating belts or through a massage will not help a person to lose weight. These are not effective in increasing endurance, or reducing weight in certain areas of the body ('spot reducing') either.

11. Sauna, steam or whirlpool baths are not effective in helping a person to reduce.

12. Fat cannot be lost from certain parts of the body, such as the abdomen, alone. Fat is lost from all over the body.

13. Special equipment and gadgets are not needed for reducing weight. They are expensive and not effective in helping a person to lose weight.

14. It is not necessary to join a club, spa or salon to do exercise for reducing weight, but a person may join for training or if it makes her want to exercise.

> **Exercise and a reducing diet will help a person lose weight and keep it off better than exercise alone or diet alone.**

IDEAS AND SUGGESTIONS FOR LEARNING ABOUT OBESITY AND WEIGHT CONTROL

What to learn	What to do	Who/what to use
Obesity can be prevented. Eating the right kinds and amounts of food and exercising can help to control obesity.	Weigh yourself, take your height and calculate your BMI (wt. in kgs/height in metres squared). What is the result? Also stand naked in front of a	Scale Measuring tape Ruler Nomogram p.185

What to learn	What to do	Who/what to use
Messages: — A person must take personal responsibility for his health and nutrition. — Part of that responsibility is knowing what contributes to poor health and nutrition and doing healthy things to prevent them.	mirror. Using your thumb and first finger try pinching the back of your arm or a fold of skin at your side or on your tummy. How wide must those fingers be to pinch? The wider they are the more the fat in that area. Get other people to do the same. Ask yourself several questions: Am I just right, too fat or too thin? Am I satisfied with the way I am? If not, what can I do? How much do I and others need to gain or lose?	
	How will I go about it? What will happen if I do not do something about being too fat? Did my parents do anything? If still alive what can they do to live longer? If dead already, why? Am I setting a good example for my children? Are we eating too much or exercising too little? When last have we had a check-up?	Nutritionist/Nutrition assistant Physical education teacher
— Obesity is a common public health problem.	Discuss with doctor, nutritionist or other qualified person who knows about sensible dieting and exercise for weight control.	People who control their weight well; yourself, and members of your family; doctor; health records; nutritionist

What to learn	What to do	Who/what to use
— Obesity can affect health in many ways. It is a major risk factor for diabetes, high blood pressure and heart attack.	List ways in which obesity affects health and discuss with people who are too fat. Do they suffer any of these?	Doctor Nutritionist Dietitian Fat people
— Healthy things to do are eating right, exercising regularly, getting enough rest, getting check-ups often.	Discuss with qualified persons in health.	Nutritionist/dietitian; nutrition assistant; doctor; physical education teacher; food guide
— Eating right means eating the right amounts of food from the six food groups and cutting back on fats, salt, sugar and alcohol.	Demonstrate food portions and combinations to make healthy meals. Give examples of foods that are high in starch and sugar (carbohydrates), fat and alcohol. Demonstrate how to prepare foods without frying.	Food composition tables; food groups charts; actual foods or pictures of foods; cooking utensils
— The best exercises help the muscles to work at will and strengthen the heart and lungs.	Demonstrate types of exercises or get a qualified person to demonstrate.	Physiotherapist Physical education teacher
— Exercises must be done regularly, hard (vigorous) and long enough to be effective.	Demonstrate types of exercises or get a qualified person to demonstrate.	Physiotherapist Physical education teacher
— When people are very fat and they lose weight, this will help to control diabetes and high blood pressure.	Discuss sensible ways to lose weight through diet and exercise. Demonstrate procedures or get someone to do the demonstration.	Exercise instructor Real foods with portions.

14

Diabetes and high blood pressure

Diabetes

Management of diabetes

High blood pressure

*Reducing the risk of high
blood pressure*

*Ideas and suggestions for learning
about diabetes and high blood pressure*

**Health
Food and Nutrition**

WHAT YOU SHOULD BE ABLE TO DO
AFTER STUDYING THIS CHAPTER

After studying this chapter you should be able to:
— identify symptoms of diabetes and high blood pressure;
— help people understand that diet and exercise are very important for the prevention and treatment of diabetes and high blood pressure;
— keep checks on people in the community who have diabetes and high blood pressure;
— see that people who have diabetes and high blood pressure eat the right foods, exercise regularly, take their medication and follow the doctor's advice.

DIABETES

Diabetes is a disease in which glucose piles up in blood. Glucose is a type of sugar which is obtained from digested food. It piles up because it is unable to get into the cells. This is why some people refer to the condition as 'having sugar'. The full name for diabetes is **diabetes mellitus.**

How does this sugar get to pile up in the blood?
When food is digested the starches and sugars (carbohydrates) change mostly to a simple sugar called glucose. So after a meal there is a lot of the sugar glucose in the blood. Normally, insulin, a substance produced by the pancreas (sweetbread) quickly moves excess glucose out of the blood into the body cells. In diabetes, the excess glucose is not removed from the blood to the cells, so it piles up in the blood. The pile up happens because the person may either not produce any insulin or is unable to use effectively the insulin provided. Thus there are two main types of diabetes.

Types of diabetes
Types I: No insulin is produced so the person must get insulin from outside the body. This type of diabetes is also called **insulin-dependent**. It is most commonly found in children, but some adults also have this type of diabetes. This type of diabetes needs very special management and close supervision. There are fewer Type I than Type II diabetics.

Type II: Insulin is produced but the body cannot use it properly so the person with Type II diabetes does not have to get insulin.

The task is to get the insulin present utilized properly. Most persons who have this type of diabetes are obese. But some people who are not obese can also have it. Two types of management are involved: one for the obese person and the other for the non-obese. Most community workers can help people to manage their Type II or **non-insulin dependent** diabetes.

> **Testing the blood for glucose is the most reliable means of confirming that a person has diabetes.**

What about sugar in the urine?
Sugar or glucose appears in the urine when the blood has so much sugar that, as the kidneys extract waste matter and water from the blood to make urine, excess glucose escapes into the urine. So sugar in the urine is a direct result of excess sugar in the blood.

Some symptoms of diabetes
A person with diabetes may:
— urinate often. This happens because more urine is produced as water is drawn from the cells to help excrete some of the sugar.
— become very thirsty and drink a lot. The loss of excess water through the urine makes one very thirsty.
— complain of a pricking, tingling or creeping sensation on the skin and may itch a lot.
— complain of blurred vision. Some people say their eyes are cloudy or dark.
— become weak and tire easily as the various parts of the body do not get enough energy and nourishment.
— lose weight in spite of normal or increased appetite. The body tries to get nourishment by using up its muscle and fat. This usually happens in Type I diabetics.

A person who has any of those symptoms, especially someone who has diabetes in his/her family and is overweight, should be checked regularly for diabetes. If diabetes is found early and controlled the person can live a long, happy, healthy and normal life.

Who gets diabetes?
Anyone can get diabetes. Persons most likely to get diabetes are:
— obese (too fat)
— females
— of African and Indian descent

— from a diabetic family
— over forty
— women who have had large babies (10-12 lbs/5-6 kilos), or have unexpectedly lost a pregnancy or get swollen feet during pregnancy or have been pregnant many times.

For example, in the Caribbean region, about 12 in every 100 persons 40 years and over have diabetes. It is more common in women than in men.

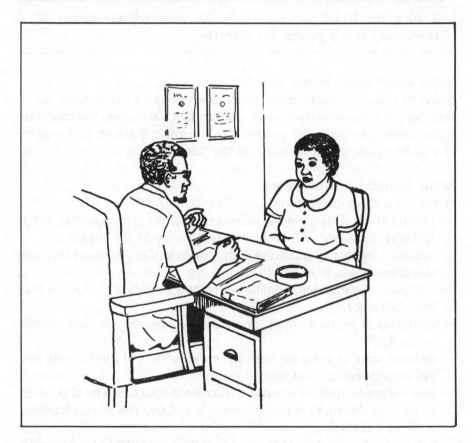

What can happen when a person has diabetes?
Diabetes can cause problems such as:
— blindness
— kidney and nerve damage
— hardening of the arteries (artherosclerosis) and heart attack
— stroke (especially when the person also has high blood pressure)
— low resistance to infections so that wounds, especially those on the feet and legs, do not heal easily. Spreading infections may cause the legs to be cut off (amputated).

> **Diabetes can be managed well or controlled so that a diabetic can have a full and satisfying life.**

Controlling diabetes means:
1. Keeping the blood sugar level normal or near normal.
2. Keeping weight down if fat.
3. Keeping blood fat low to prevent heart disease. Heart disease is nearly three times more common in diabetics than in non-diabetics.

MANAGEMENT OF DIABETES

Type I and Type II diabetes are managed differently. Type I is managed by insulin and diet. In Type II the person who is not too fat is managed by diet alone or diet plus oral drugs. The obese person is managed by weight reduction (a low-calorie diet and exercise) and oral drugs.

The diet

> **Diet is an important part of diabetic management. Each person with diabetes needs to be provided with an individualized plan, appropriate counselling in the use of the plan and follow up as necessary.**

In general, most persons with diabetes can have a normal diet based on the six food groups. The amounts of food will vary according to the amount of energy (calories) recommended for that individual. These recommendations are usually made by the doctor, with the assistance of a nutritionist or dietitian. Some doctors base total calories for children on: 1,000 calories for the first year of life and 100 additional calories for every year thereafter. So a 10-year-old child would get a diet prescription of about 1,900 calories per day while a 12-year-old would get 2,100 calories per day. As the child grows, he needs more. If he is active in sports he needs even more. Children usually have Type I diabetes and must get insulin. The diet must be balanced with the insulin type and dosage and the activity level of the child. Special, careful attention must be given to the child by his parents or guardian to help him manage his diabetes well.

For adults who are moderately active, 30 calories per kilogram (2.2 lbs) of weight are recommended. An adult who weighs about 120 lbs (54 kgs) should have about 1,600 calories per day. A pregnant woman who is diabetic will need more for the development of the baby.

Complex carbohydrate foods should form the bulk of the diet

Carbohydrates (starches, sugars), protein and fat provide calories, but it is the carbohydrates that easily provide calories. So it is recommended that 50-60% of the calories should come from complex carbohydrates. Foods such as unrefined staples (oats, whole wheat bread, corn and ground provisions), peas, beans, vegetables and fresh fruits are good sources of complex carbohydrates. They are better for the person with diabetes (and everyone) than highly refined foods such as flour, crackers, most dried and ready-to-eat cereals, sugar, honey and other sweets. Complex carbohydrates are better because they are digested slower so the sugar (glucose) from them goes into the blood more slowly, and over a longer time.

Complex carbohydrate foods also have lots of fibre. Fibre helps the body to absorb glucose slower so that the blood sugar levels are not likely to be too high. Fibre also helps a person to have regular bowel movements and to lower the fat-like substance, cholesterol, in the blood.

Persons with diabetes can have large amounts of carbohydrate but must avoid refined starchy foods and simple sugars.

The amount and type of fat

Persons who have diabetes must also watch the amount and type of fat eaten. It is recommended that about ⅓ or less (about 30%) of the total calories should come from fats. Therefore, in most cases the diabetic will have to cut back on the amount of fat eaten. Cutting back means having skimmed milk and small portions of lean meat, chicken (skin removed), fried foods (or cutting out frying altogether), 'fast foods', gravy, salad dressings, streaky bacon and avocado pear. Hard or waxy fats from meat, milk and milk products, coconut oil and red palm oil should be no more than ⅓ of the total fat eaten. These fats, together with cholesterol, help to harden and clog the blood vessels (arteries). This can lead to serious conditions such as heart attack, stroke and kidney failure. So the diabetic must also watch the amount of cholesterol eaten. Cutting back on meat portions, meat fat, eggs, whole or full cream milk, high-fat cheese, organ meats (liver, heart, kidney, tripe) and shellfish (lobster, shrimp) will help to lower the amount of cholesterol eaten.

The amount and type of protein-rich foods

Protein will provide the remaining 10-20% of the calories. Protein-rich foods, such as fish, chicken (skin removed), lean meat, low fat cheese, skimmed milk and dried peas and beans which are low in fat, are best.

FAT IN SOME FOODS

Teaspoons Fat	Portions of Food
	1 cup full cream milk
	½ cup evaporated milk
	1 rasher streaky bacon
	2 oz lean meat
	1 oz cheese
	2 oz fat meat
	2 tbsp peanut butter
	1 oz peanuts
	2 oz fish canned in oil
	5 oz pizza

Meals for Type I diabetes

In planning meals for Type I (insulin dependent) diabetes, care must be taken to include the kinds and amounts of food to get the right ratio of carbohydrate/fat/protein. In addition, food is usually divided into three meals and a bedtime snack. Sometimes there are mid-morning and mid-afternoon snacks. The meals are spaced so that the blood sugar level will be stable throughout the day. It is important for persons with Type I diabetes to eat regularly to prevent the blood sugar from getting too low or too high. The morning, noon and evening meals should contain the bulk of the calories. Meals should be taken the same time each day and should have about the same amount of food.

The planning of the diet and counselling of persons with Type I diabetes should be done by a professional person such as a dietitian, nutritionist or a doctor.

In **Type I Diabetes** management by diet is aimed at:

— reducing high blood sugar levels as well as preventing blood sugar levels from becoming too low.
— supporting the right growth and development of children who have this type of diabetes.
— preventing long-term complications (heart disease, kidney disease).
— providing all the nourishment required.

Meals for Type II diabetes

The person with Type II diabetes whose **weight is normal** should get enough calories to maintain that weight. The person should eat small amounts of food often, including a bedtime snack. This will help ensure that blood sugar levels are neither too high nor too low.

The Type II diabetic who **is obese** will need fewer calories until ideal weight is achieved. A low calorie, high fibre diet and exercise will help the person lose weight. Losing weight will usually cause the person to use the insulin available better. (See Chapter 13 — Obesity for sample meal plans and menus for moderate to low calorie meals.)

In **Type II Diabetes**, management by diet is aimed at:

— reducing weight in an obese person to make the body sensitive to available insulin.
— attaining and maintaining desirable body weight; so the obese person is given a low calorie, high fibre diet and the non-obese, normal calorie levels according to needs.
— preventing high blood sugar levels.
— preventing heart disease.
— providing all the nourishment required.

Selecting, measuring and preparing foods

Most foods provided for the rest of the family are good for the diabetic. Special dietetic foods are not necessary. Many of these foods are high in calories.

Foods To Avoid:

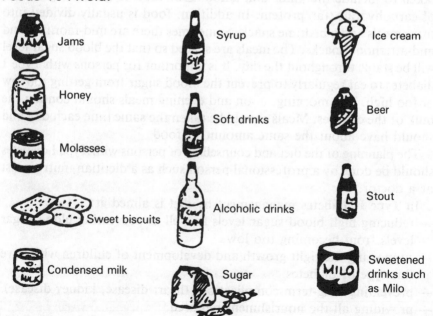

Jams

Syrup

Ice cream

Honey

Soft drinks

Beer

Molasses

Sweet biscuits

Alcoholic drinks

Stout

Condensed milk

Sugar

Sweetened drinks such as Milo

Note: ● ½ cup plain ice cream may be substituted for 1 portion staple and 2 portions fat.
   ● ½ cup jelly may be substituted for 1 portion staple.
   ● Fat allocated in diet may be used for frying.

Food for persons with diabetes should be measured. A measuring cup and a teaspoon and tablespoon are helpful. All measurements should be level, not heaped. Most foods are measured after being cooked.

In preparing foods for the diabetic, meats should be baked, boiled, roasted or broiled. Foods should not be fried or have fat added, unless fat is allowed in the meals. Vegetables may be cooked in meat broth for flavour.

Physical exercise is important for persons with diabetes

Persons with diabetes should have some form of regular physical exercise. Exercise helps the diabetic to be more sensitive to insulin so even smaller amounts of insulin are needed for the exercising muscle to take up glucose. Less insulin is required while more glucose can be stored and used. This causes the blood sugar level to be more stable in any one day.

Physical exercise also helps to reverse the resistance to insulin that occurs as a result of obesity. Exercise helps to lower blood pressure which can increase the overall problems with diabetes. The exercise should include activities such as walking briskly, riding a bicycle and swimming. The chosen activity should be carried out at least three times per week for 15-30 minutes each time.

> **Beware: Persons whose blood sugar levels are sometimes high and at other times low should avoid exercise until the blood sugar levels are normal and stable. When the levels go up and down, there will not be enough sugar stored in the muscles and liver to provide energy during exercise. The person may feel very weak and tired (fatigued). The diabetes may even worsen.**

When diabetes gets out of control

If persons with diabetes do not manage their diet properly, take enough rest and exercise or take tablets or insulin as directed, the diabetes may get out of control. When diabetes gets out of control, the person will have a 'reaction'. The blood sugar may get either too high or too low. Here's how to tell whether it is high or low and what to do.

HIGH BLOOD SUGAR	LOW BLOOD SUGAR

1. Why does it happen?

The person:	The person:
is not keeping to his/her diet	is not eating enough
is not taking regular exercise	is not eating meals and snacks at the right time
may not be getting the right dose of tablets or insulin	may be taking too much insulin or tablets for diabetes
may have an infection or fever	
may have another condition which may be affecting the body.	may be exercising without eating properly or just not exercising properly

2. How the person may feel

Thirsty	Hungry
Weak	Faint
'Bad'	Nervous
	Irritable and confused
	Drowsy

3. What may be happening to the person

Passing urine often	Having a headache
Losing appetite	Sweating a lot
Having trouble seeing properly	Trembling
Vomiting	Falling asleep
Breathing hard and heavily	

4. What the person should do

Have a drink *without sugar* Have urine tested See a doctor/nurse	Take some sugar, sweets or other form of sweet food or drink immediately.
	Get help from a doctor/nurse

What the community worker can do to help diabetics

In your work with the community you will find many people who are diabetic. Encourage them to visit the nearest clinic or health centre or their private doctor for check ups. Help them to follow their diet instructions or seek dietary counselling for them. See that they take the medicines which are prescribed. Remind and show them how to pay special attention to personal hygiene and to exercise regularly.

HIGH BLOOD PRESSURE

Blood pressure is the force of the blood against the walls of the blood vessels (arteries) which carry pure or oxygenated blood. So everyone has some blood pressure. Blood pressure can rise and fall. It can rise for a short time when a person is excited, nervous, tense, exercising or pregnant. It may become low during sleep. When a person's blood pressure remains consistently higher than normal over a long period of time, that person has high blood pressure. The condition is called hypertension or 'pressure'.

How blood pressure is measured
The pressure in the artery is measured by a special instrument called a sphygmomanometer. The instrument has a gauge on which the pressure is read. A special cuff is put around the arm. Air is pumped in until the cuff is very tight on the arm. This tightness cuts off the circulation of blood in the artery. As the air is gradually let out or released from the cuff, the pumping action of the heart shows on the gauge of the special instrument. A number is written down for that pumping force or pressure. When the heart is relaxing between beats, another number will be shown on the instrument. Both numbers represent that person's pressure. When the resting pressure remains high after several measurements, that person has high blood pressure.

Normal blood pressure
Normal blood pressure varies with age. It may be as low as 70/50 in infants or as high as 140/90 in adults. Young children and adults usually have blood pressures between 100/70 and 130/80. If an adult has a pressure of 140/90 or higher, he too has high blood pressure.

How can high blood pressure be detected?
The only way to detect high blood pressure is to have the pressure measured by a nurse, doctor or other competent health worker who has a reliable instrument.

It is important to get the blood pressure measured because very often a person has high pressure and does not even know it, until it has done

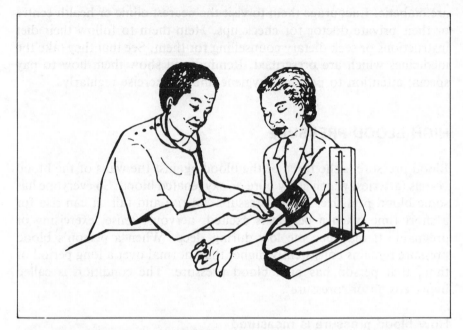

a lot of damage. This is why it is known as the 'silent disease'.

Sometimes there are symptoms such as frequent headaches, rapid heart beat, shortness of breath, weakness, dizziness, pain in the left shoulder and chest and puffy ankles (in bad cases). These symptoms may also be caused by other diseases. So the best way for a person to find out whether he has high blood pressure is to have his blood pressure measured.

What are some factors that may cause some people to get high blood pressure?

The exact cause of high blood pressure is unknown in about 90% of the cases.

There are many factors which may make some people more likely to get high blood pressure than others. Some of these are:

● **High blood pressure runs in the family**　If high blood pressure runs in the family, several members of that family may inherit the condition. We cannot do anything to change this inherited tendency but we can do other things to prevent high blood pressure.

● **Age**　Blood pressure varies with age. Any person who consistently has pressure above the limit recommended for that age has high blood pressure.

● **Eating too much salt from infancy onwards**　Breastmilk has less salt than cow's milk. Therefore, breastfeeding is an important beginning for the baby in a high-risk family. Excessive amounts of salt in the body hold water. This increases blood volume and blood pressure.

- **Being too fat** Excessive body fat places an extra demand on the heart to pump blood through more blood vessels. This increases the blood pressure.

- **The hardening of the arteries (blood vessels)** The hardening of the arteries reduces the space through which blood flows and the elasticity of the artery. If the blood cannot flow through freely, pressure builds up. Too much fat (especially the solid fats as meat and milk fat) helps to thicken the walls of the arteries. High blood pressure itself helps to harden the arteries.

- **Excessive smoking** Nicotine from tobacco stimulates the production of certain body chemicals. These chemicals raise pulse rate, blood pressure and the force of the heart's contractions.

- **Drinking too much alcohol** Excessive consumption of alcohol is associated with high blood pressure.

What can happen when a person has high blood pressure?

- When a person has high blood pressure, his heart may get larger because it has to work hard to pump blood. When it gets larger than it should be it may not be able to pump blood as well any more. Eventually it may fail to function properly. When it fails to function well, every part of the body suffers, especially the brain, kidneys and blood vessels.

- Little blisters may appear in the blood vessels in the brain. Sometimes they break suddenly and the person has a 'stroke'. There is bleeding in the brain and the person may be paralysed on one side and not able to speak, walk, eat, move about or help himself generally.

- The kidneys may be damaged. The damage is due to progressive narrowing of the blood vessels in the kidney. This reduces the amount of fluid the kidney can filter out causing a build-up of waste products in the body. Waste products 'poison' the system.

- The walls of the arteries all over the body, especially in the heart, brain and kidneys may become thick, narrowing the passage through which blood flows. This creates an extra burden on the heart as it pumps blood all over the body.

- The person may finally develop complications of the heart and blood vessels leading to heart failure, stroke and kidney damage as above. In some cases the person may not know that he/she has high blood pressure until these complications begin.

REDUCING THE RISK OF HIGH BLOOD PRESSURE

High blood pressure can be prevented. A person can reduce the risk of getting high blood pressure by:
— eating less salt and fatty foods
— keeping weight within normal range
— exercising regularly, but staying away from those exercises which involve too much effort, e.g. in moving heavy objects and lifting weight
— not having too much alcohol
— not smoking

However, if a person does have high blood pressure, he/she can reduce the risk of getting heart, kidney and blood vessel diseases by:

1. **Getting treatment early and regularly.** Part of the treatment may be special pills/medicine. He should make sure that he does not run out of the medication. He should also take his medication as directed as there may be no symptoms even though internal damage is being done. The person should have regular check-ups so that the pressure can be monitored.

2. **Reducing if too fat.** (See Chapter 13.) Weight reduction lowers pressure directly. In addition, the person will feel better, be able to exercise more and reduce his chances of a heart attack.

3. **Paying careful attention to the diet.** The person can have nutritious meals from the six food groups with more chicken, fish, and skimmed milk **rather than** fat meat, butter, full cream milk, eggs and bacon. He needs to eat less high-fat, high cholesterol and salty foods. Cholesterol is a fat-like substance found in animal sources of food, such as eggs, meat and milk fat, butter, shrimp, lobster, liver and tripe.

   Some foods to avoid because of salt are:
   Red herring
   Salt mackerel
   Salted nuts, chips
   Dried soup mixes
   Bottled sauces, pickles
   Pickled and corned meat
   Bacon, ham, sausages   These also contain lots of fat and
   Frankfurters, cheese   the fat-like substance cholesterol
   'Fast foods'   which contribute to the hardening
                                 of the arteries.

TEASPOONS SALT IN SOME FOODS

1 oz Saltfish	1
1 packet dried Soup Mix (cup-a-soup)	¼-½
2 oz Corned Beef	¼
2 oz Ham	¼
1 Frankfurter	¼
1 tablespoon Soy Sauce	½
1 oz Cheese	¼

4. **Exercising regularly.** (See Chapter 13.) Regular exercise reduces high blood pressure.

5. **Not smoking.** Cigarette smoking makes the heart need more oxygen. At the same time it reduces the amount of oxygen that is available. It also helps to increase the substances that clog up or harden the arteries. So when the pressure is already high and arteries damaged, smoking can help to bring on poor circulation, heart attack and even sudden death.

6. **Not drinking too much alcohol.** Even low alcohol consumption is associated with increased blood pressure. When heavy drinkers give up alcohol, their blood pressure is reduced.

7. **Not relying on home remedies.** Home remedies may only mask the symptoms not cure the condition.

What the community worker can do
The community worker can:
— help the person to get blood pressure checked. If high blood pressure is present, help the person to get a treatment plan from a doctor.

— focus on prevention. Involve parents, older children, teachers, sports organizations and the health team in getting children to eat well and exercise regularly.

— encourage sensible, regular exercise as part of normal life.

— help to promote exercise in the community.

— create awareness of the extent of the problem, what it can do and how it can be prevented.

— stress the importance of not smoking, reducing salt and fat intake in the diet, and losing weight if too fat.

IDEAS AND SUGGESTIONS ABOUT LEARNING ABOUT DIABETES AND HIGH BLOOD PRESSURE

What to learn	What to do	Who/what to use
— There are two types of diabetes each of which requires a different kind of management.	Read the information provided and discuss with persons who have the disease and those who treat them.	Doctor, nurse, persons with diabetes, nutritionist, dietitian, publications.
— A person with diabetes can eat many different kinds of food from regular family meals.	Show the kinds of foods people with diabetes can eat and in what amounts.	Books on meal planning for diabetics.
— A person with Type I diabetes must get insulin and must eat to match the amount and type of insulin.	Discussion with doctor/nutritionist, dietitian and diabetics on insulin.	Doctor, nurse, nutritionist, dietitian.
— Eating the same amount at the same time each day is very important for the person with Type I diabetes.	Demonstrate sample meals and snacks, foods to avoid and foods which can be substituted for each other.	Real foods, sample meals, foods with high, medium and low fat and sugar.
— Different complications happen to a person with diabetes if the condition is not controlled (e.g. blindness, nerve damage).	Get people with diabetes who have and have not controlled their condition well to share their experiences.	People who have and have not controlled their condition well.

What to learn	What to do	Who/what to use
— Control means keeping the blood sugar level normal or near normal.	Discuss with doctor and persons who have maintained good control of their sugar levels.	Doctor, other people.
— When diabetes is out of control, the blood sugar may get too high or too low. Both situations are dangerous.	Review with group the procedures to follow if sugar level is too high or too low.	Charts/leaflets, members of the group.
— Ways to control high blood pressure are: eating less salt, keeping weight within normal limits, avoiding alcohol, avoiding smoking.	Suggest foods people with high blood pressure should not have and explain why. Give examples of foods which are high in salt/sodium. Discuss the effects of alcohol and smoking with the group.	Real foods or pictures of foods high in salt; amount of salt (in teaspoons) in some foods; doctor.
— Foods can be seasoned well without salt.	Prepare some dishes and taste. Have others taste too.	Herbs and spices such as ginger, pimento (allspice), cloves, rosemary, French thyme and garlic; citrus juice; prepared dishes and utensils for tasting; recipe books.
— High blood pressure can be prevented.	List and discuss with doctor and community members, ways to prevent high blood pressure.	Doctor, community members.
— If medication is a part of treatment for high blood pressure the person must have it all the time as advised by his doctor.	List and discuss with doctor and community members, ways to prevent high blood pressure.	Doctor, community members.

What to learn	What to do	Who/what to use
— Many people apply home remedies for diabetes and high blood pressure (hypertension), but it is not wise to do this.	Find out from people what they do to keep their diabetes and high blood pressure under control and discuss the dangers of relying on home treatments/'cures'. Encourage them to use the health services.	People with diabetes and high blood pressure.

15

Improving health and nutrition in the community

How to protect children against diseases

Malnutrition and infection

Child spacing

Keeping watch

Correcting wrong beliefs about food and nutrition

Producing foods at home

Health
Food and Nutrition
Agriculture

What you should be able to do
after studying this chapter

After studying this Chapter, you should be able to:
— understand why immunization is important.
— explain to mothers/childminders that children who are not immunized can get infections.
— explain to mothers/childminders that children need a certain number of vaccines to protect them fully from each disease.
— show mothers how malnutrition and infection are related.
— advise mothers when to get their children immunized.
— identify persons who need family planning.
— show why family planning is important.
— know why food supplies and health should be watched.
— help people to correct wrong beliefs about food and nutrition.
— encourage families to produce some of the foods they need.
— advise families where they can get information on how to produce food.

HOW TO PROTECT CHILDREN AGAINST DISEASES

Many diseases are spread by germs which can cause infection. Germs are so small that we cannot see them with our naked eyes. They are around us everywhere; in the air, in water, in nearly everything we touch and even on our skin. Some germs are harmless, but others are harmful and attack the body.

Dangerous germs can pass from one person to another in different ways. If someone has a disease in his chest or throat, he coughs. When he coughs, germs go into the air. The germs may then be breathed in by someone else and cause that person to have the same disease. Tuberculosis and measles are passed on in this way.

If someone has diarrhoea, he may pass many germs or parasites in his stools. If the stools get into water and someone drinks this water, that person may also get diarrhoea. Germs from stools are most often passed on by unwashed hands. Anyone who looks after children should be particularly careful to wash their hands after going to the toilet, after changing the baby's nappies, or after doing anything else which brings the hands into contact with stools.

These diseases which are passed from person to person are called infectious diseases. They are sometimes called '**communicable diseases**', meaning that they can be passed on to others.

MALNUTRITION AND INFECTION

The most common kinds of disease in children are malnutrition and infections. A child with malnutrition is not properly nourished because he does not eat enough of the right foods. A child with an infection has harmful organisms (germs) growing inside his body. These germs make him sick. Many children are malnourished and also suffer from some type of infection. Children who are malnourished cannot fight germs well. They often get very ill and may die. Breastfeeding, proper weaning, eating enough of the right foods and immunization help to increase a child's resistance to infectious diseases.

If a child has a strong resistance to germs, his body can fight them well. The germs will not easily make him ill. There are two ways of making sure that a child builds up a strong resistance to germs:
— proper feeding
— immunization.

Proper feeding nourishes the body well and makes the child strong. If a child has an infection, it helps prevent the infection from getting worse. Diarrhoea is much less serious in children who are well nourished and they get diarrhoea much less often than the under-nourished child.

If a mother breastfeeds her newborn baby, she builds up his resistance against germs. By giving this perfect baby-food she also improves his nutrition. The milk she gives him contains special substances so that the baby will not get infection from germs. The baby will be protected against these germs for at least three months. At three months baby should then be immunized against certain diseases.

Immunization is done by giving children special medicines called vaccines. The vaccines are given by injection or by mouth.

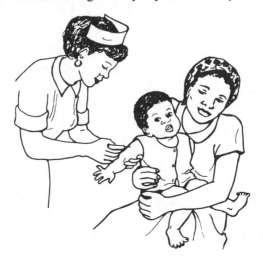

Why immunization is necessary

Immunization gives protection against some dangerous diseases which can cause much sickness and death among babies and young children. The immunizations given in the health centres protect babies from six dangerous diseases:

DISEASES YOUNG CHILDREN MAY GET	
Name of disease	**What it causes**
Tuberculosis	May attack any part of the body but usually attacks the lung. It causes severe coughing, loss of appetite, loss of weight and weakness.
Polio	Is a serious disease. The person with polio has a high fever, severe headache and diarrhoea. Polio sometimes causes parts of the body to become paralyzed.
Diphtheria	Attacks the throat and causes suffocation and death.
Pertussis (Whooping Cough)	Causes distressing coughing, vomiting and weakness.
Tetanus (Lock Jaw)	Causes painful spasms of the muscles of the face. These spasms spread throughout the body. The person cannot eat. He may die.
Measles	Attacks the whole body including the inside of the mouth. It causes high fever, a rash and coughing. There may be severe complications such as pneumonia and diarrhoea. He may also lose his appetite and become malnourished.

To be fully protected against these serious diseases, children must have the full course of vaccines at the right ages. The following chart shows how this should be done:

IMMUNIZATION CHART

Age at which immunization given	Diseases immunization prevents	Name of vaccine	How it is given	What happens after
Birth 3 months	Tuberculosis	BCG	Injection under skin	After 3-4 weeks a small lump comes up where the needle went in. It may burst and drain water for a few weeks.
3 months	Diphtheria Pertussis (Whooping cough) Tetanus (Lock jaw)	DPT	Injection under skin	May cause red, sore arm and fever for about one day. Parents should be told that this may happen. They should be advised to give the baby half an aspirin tablet in some milk or water.
	Polio	TOPV	By mouth — a few drops put on the back of the tongue or on a lump of Sugar.	

Age at which immunization given	Diseases immunization prevents	Name of vaccine	How it is given	What happens after
5 months	2nd DPT + 2nd Polio	DPT + TOPV	Injection under skin By mouth — a few drops put on the back of the tongue or on a lump of sugar.	May cause red, sore arm and fever for about one day. Parents should be told that this may happen. They should be advised to give the baby half an aspirin tablet in some milk or water.
7 months	3rd DPT + 3rd Polio	DPT + TOPV	Injection under skin By mouth — a few drops put on the back of the tongue or on a lump of Sugar.	May cause red, sore arm and fever for about one day. Parents should be told that this may happen. They should be be advised to give the baby half an aspirin tablet in some milk or water.
9-15 months	Measles + Rubella	M - R	One injection under skin	If it is not given before 1 year, the child may get measles after the

Age at which immunization given	Diseases immunization prevents	Name of vaccine	How it is given	What happens after
				immunization. Sometimes there is a little fever about 7 days after the vaccination. This soon goes away.
4-5 years or before school entrance		Mantoux Test*	One injection under skin	If a red patch develops, the child is all right. If it does not, he will need to be given the BCG vaccine again.
		DPT 'Booster' Shot	One drop on the tongue	
		TOPV 'Booster' Shot	One drop on the tongue	

* The Mantoux Test is an injection given under the skin. It will test whether the BCG vaccine given at birth — 3 months is working.

It is important to know that one injection is not enough to protect babies against these diseases. They must be given the full course of three injections of DPT and three doses of TOPV, at three months, five months and seven months, respectively.

How to keep vaccines safely

Vaccines have to be stored and handled with care. They can be spoilt if they get too hot or are exposed to the sun. Measles, BCG and polio vaccines are the most sensitive and should be kept frozen. DPT vaccine should not be frozen but it should be kept cool. Vaccines are expensive.

Keeping vaccines cool in a refrigerator or cooler

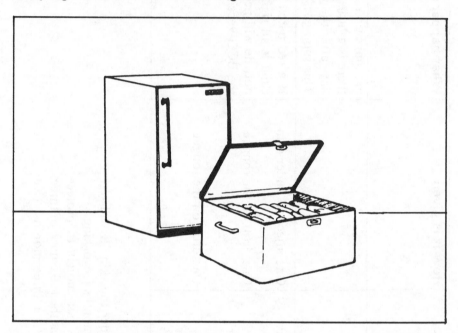

What the community worker can do

It takes a lot of time and work but an immunization programme is a vital part of Primary Health Care. It is also a good activity for involving the community.

The community worker is very important in an immunization programme. She should:

1. Involve the family and community in immunization programmes.
2. Explain that it is important to immunize children in the community.
3. Get community leaders to see that it is a good idea.
4. Let community leaders help her to find all the children who need immunization.
5. Get parents/childminders to take children to the health centre.
6. Help get the children to the immunization centres at the right time on the correct day.
7. Teach mothers the importance of keeping immunization cards clean and bringing them to the clinic each time.

CHILD SPACING

Child spacing means having children far enough apart so that they will be properly cared for. Having too many children too often can be a burden on the parents. Also, a mother can become sick if she has too many children too often.

Good child spacing makes for better health and general well being of mother, child and family.

Where people can learn about child spacing

People can learn about child spacing at the following places: hospital clinic; health centre or clinic; rural maternity centre; family planning clinic; private doctor.

What the community worker can do about encouraging proper child spacing

There are several things the community worker can do to encourage good child spacing:
— Help people understand the importance of child spacing.
— Find out the persons in the community best qualified to give family planning advice.
— Know the location of the nearest family planning centre and the clinic hours.
— Identify persons who need family planning services.
— Send people who want to learn about family planning to the right place.

The community worker should set a good example of being a responsible parent. Practising proper child spacing is as important as helping others to space their children.

HOW CHILD SPACING IS RELATED TO HEALTH AND NUTRITION

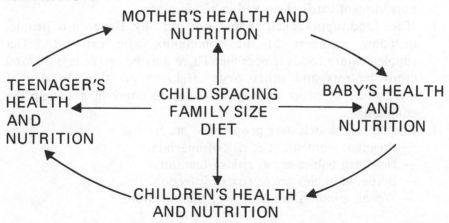

KEEPING WATCH

An experienced mother knows how to keep watch over her young children so as to make sure they are safe. She watches against falls, burns, cuts, dirty or dangerous things being put in the mouth and other accidents which may happen. She probably watches her baby while still going about her daily work. This 'keeping watch' is called 'surveillance'.

We can watch over the nutrition of a young child through seeing him regularly and through keeping a growth chart (see page 130). A growth chart can be a useful warning sign. As soon as the child stops growing well we can see this on the growth chart.

It is just as important to keep watch over the nutrition of a community. This is so that we can tell beforehand if anything is starting to go wrong. We can tell if people's nutrition is getting worse, if more children are getting diarrhoea, if more people are getting anaemia or if food is becoming short. If we find that something is going wrong with the nutrition of the community, we can do something about it. What is important is to find out early.

Keeping watch over the community means keeping records. That is why the nurse asks for information on the growth of all the children under her care, on new births or deaths of patients who attend the health centre and on cases of some illnesses. These records will show how many cases of a particular illness there are, and if the cases are increasing, the nurse must find out why. If cases are decreasing, health workers can feel proud that their work is well done.

Here are some of the things the community worker can do when 'keeping watch'.

1. Encourage mothers/childminders to get birth certificates of the children in their care and keep them safely.
2. Remind them to get their children immunized and keep their appointment cards clean and in a safe place.
3. If the food supply is getting low, find out why. Report it to people, including members of the community who can help. Get supplementary foods if possible. There may be severe loss of food crops by rats and other pests. Help to get the Ministry of Agriculture or other appropriate body to come in and help the community.
4. Keep special watch over people who are 'at risk':
   — Pregnant women are at risk of anaemia.
   — Newborn babies are at risk of tentanus.
   — Bottlefed babies are at risk of infection.
   — Weaning babies are at risk of malnutrition.

— Low birth weight babies are at risk of malnutrition.
— Very poor families are at risk of malnutrition.

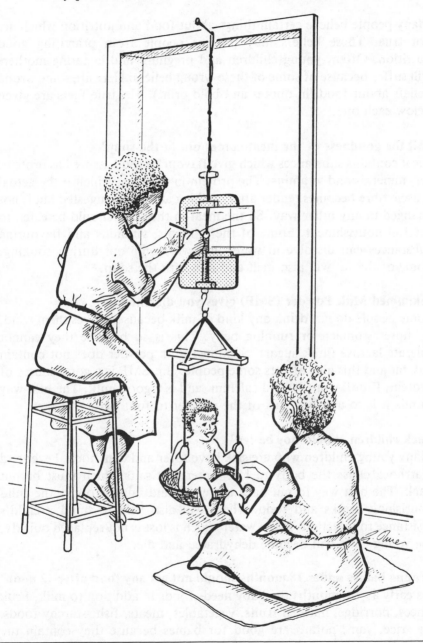

Community workers must keep watch and look out for trouble before it comes
   Prevention is better than cure!

CORRECTING WRONG BELIEFS ABOUT FOOD AND NUTRITION

Many people believe certain things about food and nutrition which are not true. These beliefs may prevent people from practising good nutrition. Often, young children and pregnant and lactating mothers will suffer because of some of these wrong beliefs. Here are some wrong beliefs about food (in quotes and bold print). The true facts are given below each one.

'All the goodness of the meat comes out in the soup'
Meat contains substances which give flavour to food, as well as protein, fat, minerals and vitamins. The protein in the meat which is the actual muscle fibre becomes tender after cooking and easily digested but is not changed in any other way. So the meat in the soup should be eaten to get full nourishment. Some of the minerals, vitamins and flavouring substances can dissolve in water and will come out during cooking. Some of the fat will also melt and mix with the soup.

'Skimmed Milk Powder (SMP) gives you diarrhoea'
Some people do not drink any kind of milk because it gives them wind, an upset stomach or running belly. This is so because they cannot tolerate lactose (milk sugar). Skimmed milk powder does not contain any fat and this also affects some people. But SMP is a good source of protein, Riboflavin (B_2) and calcium, and is a good milk. The best way to mix it is to add one part of the powder to four parts of water.

'Sick children should not be fed'
Many young children who are sick have fever and diarrhoea. Fever and diarrhoea cause the body to lose water and salts which must be put back. The best way to put back the water and salts is to give the child nourishing drinks and food. These will also help to build a child's resistance to infection. If the water which is lost is not replaced quickly, the young child will become dehydrated and die.

'Young babies under 18 months should not get any food after 12 noon'
As early as 4-6 months the baby needs foods in addition to milk. Fruit juices, porridge, mashed fruits, vegetables, meats, fish, starchy foods, e.g. rice, yam, potato are good for babies because they contain the nourishment they need to grow and develop well. These foods should be given in small amounts, at first around mid-morning and mid-afternoon. From about 9 months of age, when the child should be eating from the 'family pot', he should get three main meals each day to

fit in with the family's eating pattern. So afternoon and evening meals are important.

'Liver makes the baby's tongue heavy'

Liver is a very good source of protein, iron and vitamins A and B. These are all necessary for good growth and to keep the body healthy. Liver and other good foods will not prevent the baby from talking when he is ready.

'Good food will kill a malnourished child'

The malnourished child, even more than a healthy well-fed child, needs good nourishing foods to help him grow, develop and live a normal life. Feeding him highly nutritious foods often is important if he is to get well again. After he is better he should continue getting nourishing foods often, and in larger quantities as he grows older. Good food keeps young children alive and well.

'Too much rice will cause you to be light in weight'

Rice is a starchy food which gives energy to the body. It contains a little protein. Brown rice contains some of the B vitamins. Three parts of rice to one part of peas makes a good-quality nourishing dish, even without meat added. Eating too much rice will make a person heavy, not light, espeically if he does not use up plenty of energy by being active.

'If you have an ulcer (e.g. on the foot) do not eat rice, fish, ripe banana, or avocado pear as they will give bad blood and cause the sore to worsen'

When we speak about 'bad blood' we mean that it does not have enough iron. Iron is found in molasses, liver, kidney, heart, dried beans and green leafy vegetables. So to keep our blood healthy, we should eat plenty of these foods. Good food is important for ulcers to heal quickly.

'Bush tea warms the stomach and takes the rawness off the chest'

The stomach is securely tucked away and is always warm. Bush tea, or any other hot drink will not make it any warmer. Bush tea should never replace a good, nutritious breakfast for the young child.

'If a woman is breastfeeding and gets into a temper, or becomes hot from working in the sun or from ironing, her milk will become sour and is not good for the baby'

Breast milk is the best food for the baby. If a breastfeeding mother is contented, well-nourished and gets enough rest, her body will produce enough breast milk for her baby. This milk is always pure, fresh, nourishing and at the right temperature. Nothing a woman does will affect the quality of the milk.

'Health Foods will keep you healthy'

Some foods which are termed 'health foods' are: yogurt, irish moss (sea moss), vinegar and honey. These foods (which are usually very expensive) are no more nutritious than a good diet of foods from each of the food groups. We should not pay high prices for foods just because they are called 'health foods'. There is no need to make vitamin pills or tonics a part of the daily diet unless they are prescribed by a doctor.

PRODUCING FOODS AT HOME

Many families feed themselves well from what they produce. No matter how small the space, each family can try to grow foods or rear small stock which will help to nourish their bodies. Foods produced at home

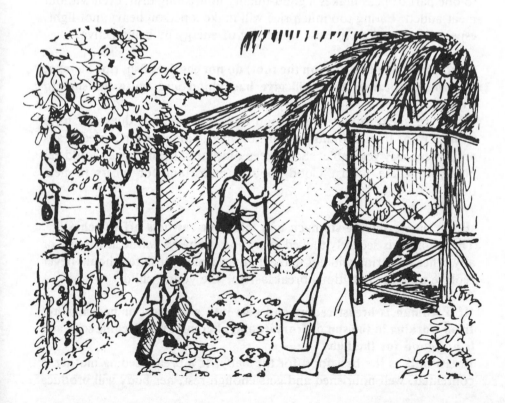

will cost less than foods which are bought in the market and will be fresh and good tasting. Some of the foods can also be sold and the money used to buy foods which cannot be produced at home.

A home garden may be a large or small plot of land, one or two beds, or a hillside slope. Where there is not enough land to cultivate (as in the town), gardens may be planted in old pots, old car tyres, large bamboos or gasolene drums cut in half across or lengthwise.

Small domestic animals like goats, chickens, rabbits and pigeons can also be reared even if there is not enough land space. They can be put in pens and cages and fed on cut grass and other feeds.

There are many good reasons for producing food at home. Some of these are:
— Good use can be made of waste land areas.
— Clearing the waste land rids the place of insect pests, slugs, mice, rats and weeds.
— Nutritious, tasty and cheap foods can be provided.
— Money is saved by not having to buy expensive foods in the market.
— Families earn money by selling the extra food that they cannot eat.
— Foods can be had fresh at any time. (Peas and beans can be dried and stored for later use.)
— Manure from animals and waste from the kitchen can be used to keep the soil in good condition.
— Family members get good exercise in gardening and looking after animals.
— Fuel (biogas) can be produced from animal droppings to cook foods. In some cases the fuel can run small farm machinery or provide light for a chicken house.

How to get the best returns from the family garden and farm
— The soil should be prepared and manured well before planting.
— Good quality seeds and plants should be used.
— Animals reared should be healthy and productive.
— There should be enough water for vegetables and good quality feeds for animals.
— Plants should be put where they can get plenty of sunshine.
— Gardens and animal pens or cages should be kept clean.
— Plants and animals should be watched to find out if anything is going wrong so that it can be corrected quickly.
— All family members should take part. The cost of labour will be less. Children can be taught to grow the foods they eat and enjoy and old people can get much needed exercise.
— The Agricultural Extension Officer or other suitable person should be asked for advice on crop and animal care.

Some nourishing foods to produce

Staples (cereals): maize or sorghum
Legumes/nuts: beans, groundnuts, coconuts
Vegetables: carrots, okra, pumpkin, spinach, tomatoes, cabbage, sweet peppers
Food from animals: meat (rabbits, goats, chickens, pigeons, ducks); eggs, milk
Fruits: orange, mangoes, tangerines, grapefruit, guava, avocado (pear)

Drying foods

Some foods can be dried for later use, for example, groundnuts and beans which can be used for eating as well as planting. Drying helps foods to keep their nourishment and flavour. Many foods need no special preparation before drying. Here are hints for sun-drying foods.

● Select high-quality, fresh produce, all at the same degree of ripeness or maturity.

● Sort grains and clean away trash, dirt and grit.

● Wash fruits and vegetables. Peel carefully, if necessary, with a stainless steel knife to prevent darkening of cut surfaces.

● Slice or chop fruits and vegetables into small pieces.

● Blanch vegetables to destroy enzymes or chemical substances that cause spoilage. To blanch: put the chopped foods in a strainer, colander or open-weave cloth bag and plunge into boiling water. Hold for 1-2 minutes. Drain quickly and then steep in cold water to cool. Drain and put to dry, spreading evenly in thin layers.

● Dry on trays (meshed bottom, if possible) in a dust-free area. Place trays on a frame or stand so that air can circulate and also to keep the food away from flies and dirt. It is also important to cover the trays with mosquito netting or an empty tray turned upside down to protect the food from flies or dust. Stir the food or turn periodically to speed up drying.

● Dry some products, such as green vegetables, in the shade, where air can circulate freely.

No special equipment and little labour are needed to dry foods in the sun. However, this may take a long time. Also, when foods are sun-dried in the open they stand a chance of getting wet by rain. This causes them to become mouldy and spoil.

Solar driers are becoming popular. They are very handy for protecting the foods from dirt, rain and animals. Foods are dried faster and moulds and germs are killed in the drying process. Special equipment is required for solar drying. For information on how to build solar driers ask the Agricultural Extension Officer in your area.

Solar Drier — Front View

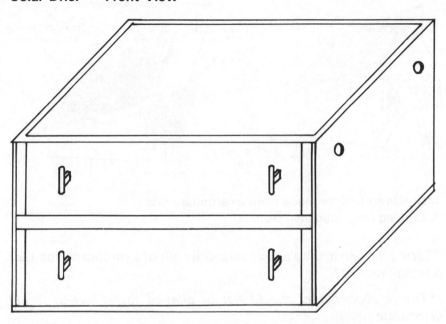

Solar Drier — Inside View

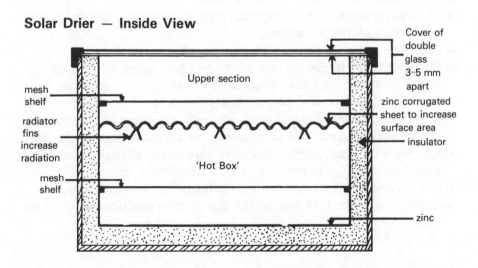

A solar drier can be made from wood or cardboard, to any reasonable size. The bottom and sides are usually insulated to keep in the heat. The inner part is painted flat black (to absorb the heat of the sun), and the top is covered with clear plastic, fibre glass or glass (to let the sun into the cabinet). It also has inlet and outlet holes for air and water vapour respectively.

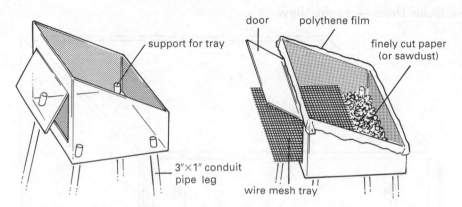

A simple solar drier made from a cardboard box.
A wooden box could also be used

Here is how to make a simple solar drier out of a cardboard box.(See diagram above)**

The cardboard drier should not be allowed to get wet as it will deteriorate rapidly.

- Get a cardboard box of standard size.
- Cut away a portion of the top slantingly to about one-half the height of the box on the lower end.
- Paint the inside of the box black.
- Make six holes in the bottom of the box and insert 3-inch (7.5 cm) pieces of 1-inch (2.5 cm) diameter PVC conduit (to serve as legs, ventilation ducts and support for drying tray).
- Place clean sawdust, dried grass or finely cut paper on the bottom of the box. These act as an insulator to keep the heat in the box.
- Fit a piece of clean, sturdy, fine mesh wire on top of the PVC conduit above the sawdust in the box. This is the drying tray.
- Cover the top of the box with clear polythene (plastic) film.
- Cut a door in the rear wall of the box to load and unload foods on mesh tray.

Care of the solar drier
- Place the solar drier in the open air well away from the house roof to prevent rain water from falling on the drier.
- Change the insulation in the drier regularly.
- Fumigate or disinfect the drier after drying each type of food crop.
- Check for leaks, wood-worms and termites in wooden driers. If these are found, treat and repair the box.

For the wooden drier you will need:
- Tools:
  saw, plane, rule or tape, pencil or chalk, set square
- Materials (except insulator): [Dimension — 2′ 6″ × 2′ 6″ (0.75 × 0.75 metres)]
  ½ sheet ½″-¾″ (1.25-2.90 cm) plyboard or pieces of other suitable boards
  1½ lbs 2″ or 1½″ (0.7 kilos, 5 cm or 3.75 cm) nails
  1½ yds (1.4 metres) chicken wire
  ½ yd (0.5 metres) fine mesh wire
  ½″-1″ (1.25-2.5 cm) diameter PVC pipe
  1 quart (litre) flat black paint
  1 quart (litre) coloured paint (outer portion) or flat black paint
  2 yds (metres) plastic or polythene sheeting
  1 pair 2″ (5 cm) hinges and bolts
- Insulating materials:
  sawdust, bagasse, dried grass

To build the wooden solar drier:
1. Cut and plane the board if necessary.
2. Construct the frame and floor the bottom.
3. Put in the walls.
4. Cut the boards for the double floor and put them in place without nailing them down. Mark outlet holes and cut them through both floors.
5. Put in the desired insulating materials and nail down the second floor. Next insert the PVC pipe through the holes.
6. Construct the door at the rear wall, putting on the hinges.
7. Cut outlet holes at the top of the side walls. Put fine mesh wire to cover holes from outside.
8. Paint the inside black, and if desired, the outside too, using flat black paint.
9. Put on the top — either plastic, glass or fibreglass. Put strips of wood to secure the plastic top and add a neat finish. Allow about an inch space at the bottom and at the top for water to run off in times of rainfall.
10. Secure the door with bolts.
11. Paint the outlet portion and allow to dry.

The top of the cabinet reclines at a slightly sloping angle to allow water to run off.

SUGGESTIONS FOR PRODUCING SOME FOODS*

Chickens

— Rear home-hatched chickens or rear day-old ones which can be bought from the Agricultural Society or other grain stores.
— Keep chickens in safe coops where rats and dogs will not get at them.
— Feed them well. Give them clean water in clean vessels.
   They are ready for eating in 8-12 weeks and for laying in 5-6 months.

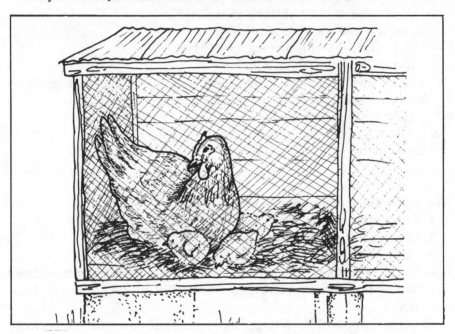

Rabbits

— Make a strong, comfortable hutch where rats and dogs cannot get at the rabbits.
— Make separate troughs for water and feeds.
— Get healthy, good breeds of animals. Feed them well. Handle them carefully. Keep the hutch and surroundings clean.
— Watch for signs of illness and treat or seek help from the Agricultural Extension Officer or the Young Farmers' Clubs.
   Rabits are ready for eating when they are 8-12 weeks old. If properly managed they can produce 3 sets of young rabbits per year.
   Rabbits also provide skins (hides) for craft items and manure for gardens.

* Adapted from Ministry of Agriculture, Jamaica.

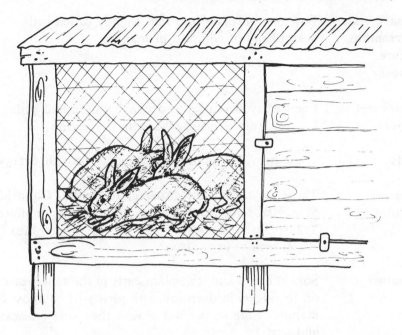

Good crops to grow in the back yard or garden.

These are nutritious and easy to grow with little effort either in the rains or the dry season if you can water them.

Legumes These enrich the soil and do not need much compost or manure.

Groundnuts Grow on ridges or mounds. A deep soil is needed. Plant early in the rains, harvest and dry under cover.

Beans/cowpeas Grow in flat beds. As with groundnuts, plant early in the rains, harvest and dry pods under cover.

Green leafy and yellow vegetables These provide vitamins, iron and fibre.

Pumpkins, melons & related varieties Dig a hole, fill with topsoil and compost or manure, plant seeds or transplant seedlings in it.

Carrots Plant in rows on slightly raised beds. They are good raw or cooked.

Spinach/Kale/ Amaranthus/ Lettuce/ Cabbage	Sow or transplant into flat, slightly raised beds with plenty of compost or manure.
Okra/sweet pepper	Plant early in rains into deep, slightly raised beds. Protect from termites. Water in dry season.
Fruits	These provide vitamins and bananas provide energy.
Pawpaw/ Bananas	These are the fastest growing tree crops. Dig a big hole, fill with topsoil and compost or manure. Transplant seedlings (or banana side shoots) into it. Water well in dry season.
Tomatoes	Sow in boxes and transplant early in the rainy season on to ridges, in deep soil with plenty of compost or manure. Late in the wet season they suffer disease and pests.
Staples	These provide energy, and maize has protein and vitamins too.
Maize	Sow on ridges, or on flat watered beds in the dry season. Use plenty of manure or compost. It is a good idea to grow maize and beans or groundnuts together on the same ridges.
Yams, Sweet potatoes	Grow on big mounds made of topsoil. Use a stake for the vine to climb up.
Cassava	Grow from cuttings early in the rains. Although lacking protein and vitamins, cassava can be left to survive the dry season and to fend for itself for up to two years, and the tubers dug up when required.

COPING WITH DISASTERS

In times of disaster such as after hurricanes, storms, floods, earthquakes and fires, people in the community may need special attention. They may need food, clothes, shelter, medical and nursing care and other help urgently. Safe drinking water and food may become scarce. Poor sanitation may increase numbers of rats, flies and other disease carriers. Many people may be at risk of infections, disease and malnutrition.

Every family member needs special care and attention, but especially children, pregnant and lactating women, the old and the disabled, diabetics and the mentally ill. These groups of people must be fed, kept clean, warm and secure. People who are on medication, such as those with high blood pressure, should have a good supply of tablets so that they do not 'run out' when roads are blocked or if it rains for several days.

HELP PEOPLE PLAN AHEAD

● How are they going to take care of members of their family with special needs?
● Where are they going for refuge if their roof blows off?
● How are they going to keep their bottled, canned and dried foods clean, dry and safe?
● How will they replace old stocks of food and water with fresh ones as often as they can to ensure a safe supply when disaster strikes?
● How will they make sure they have enough food, water, fuel and other supplies to last them for a week or two? Part of that emergency store should be foods families have preserved themselves such as dried peas and beans, yams, cassava, flours made from root and tree crops, corned and pickled meat and/or fish, dried fruit, vinegar, jams, jellies and chutney.

Foods to shop for as part of the emergency store include:
(a) Staples — cereals such as rice, cornmeal, flour, crackers, oats.
(b) Concentrated energy source — such as fat, condensed milk.
(c) Source of protein — canned meats, fish, eggs, canned and dried beans, peanuts and dried milk.

It will be easier on the family if each time they shop they buy one or two items that will go into the emergency store. Buy foods that will store for some time without spoiling and will not be too bulky for cupboard or other storage space. The days following a storm or earthquake are times for food that is easy to prepare and serve.

Here is an idea of how much food a family of six members — an elderly lady, two middle-aged adults (male and female), two teenagers (boy and girl) and a 7-9 year old school child will need to store to last for a week.

5½ kilos	12 lbs	rice
5½ kilos	12 lbs	flour
1 kilo	2 lbs	crackers

1 kilo	2 lbs	oats
5½ kilos	12 lbs	maize flour
½ kilo	1 lb	milk powder
6 (14 oz) cans		condensed milk
3 (12 oz) cans		corned beef
6 (3½ oz) cans		sardines and/or mackerel
½ kilo	1 lb	dried, salted fish
½ kilo	1 lb	dried peas
1 litre	1 quart	cooking oil
2½ kilos	5½ lbs	sugar
4 (20 oz) cans		fruit juice

If the family cured yam, cassava flour, potatoes, corned meat or fish, and made jams and jellies, they can cut back on purchased cereals, canned meat and fish and sugar. That's why it is wise to preserve foods.

When buying food for emergency stores, bear in mind that there may be a shortage of electricity and piped water for several days at a time. Some of what the family buys should be usable without refrigeration or cooking. This includes canned meat, fish, fruit, milk, vegetables, juices as well as biscuits, peanuts, condensed milk, packaged oats as included in the sample above.

Foods that the family likes and enjoys should be on hand. It is also a good idea for the family to keep handy a supply of sugar, salt (6-10 lbs), spice, vinegar and seasoning so that they can pickle fresh meat, chicken or fish so that they will not spoil readily.

Fuel for lighting and cooking must also be on hand so the family should have in reserve a bag of charcoal and 2-3 gallons of kerosene even if these are not their regular cooking fuel. A one- or two-burner kerosene stove and a charcoal stove are excellent stand-by cookers.

Households should store **water** too. Whatever the natural mishap, public water supplies are exposed to damage or interruption. When public water supply systems are damaged, families are in danger from disease germs which may enter broken water pipes.

Households should have some container where water for several days' drinking, cooking, and dishwashing and bathing needs can be stored out of reach of flies, cockroaches and mice. For a family of six (three adults and three children) two or three 4-gallon plastic buckets with tightly-fitting covers can provide adequate drinking water. For other purposes, one or two 40-gallon plastic or galvanized drums would be ideal. In places where water pressure in piped systems is not reliable, households should keep these vessels full at all times.

WHEN DISASTER STRIKES

● **Have enough water and keep it safe.**
Whenever there is warning of bad weather, storage vessels should be washed and filled with clean water. To maintain a supply of clean water, containers should be kept covered, clean utensils should be used to take water from pails or drums and drinking water should be boiled for **at least five minutes**. Sometimes fuel is a problem, in which case families should use water purification tablets sold by pharmacies and generally distributed by government relief agencies after hurricanes and other disturbances. It is important that the tablets are used at the rate recommended, that is, four tablets per gallon of water. Two drops of household bleach per gallon of water will also help to keep water safe. Rain water caught in clean containers is also safe for all household needs.

● **Use foods carefully and creatively.**
In times of disaster concentrate on the staples, peas and beans, food from animal sources and a source of fat. If the family has a farm, a chicken, pig or goat may be so badly injured that it must be prepared for the pot without delay. What the family cannot consume immediately must be preserved well to prevent spoilage and ill health. (See method for pickling/curing meat — Annex 5.)

The family may have to use the available canned or corned meat or fish, eggs, cheese, milk (especially powdered milk), maize flour, rice, flour and what they can get of the provisions — green banana, plantain and potato, dried coconut and cooking oil and margarine, and fruits which are blown off the trees. Fresh vegetables such as cabbage and carrots and spinach may be in short supply so they may have to do without them or buy canned substitutes as their means permit or they can sprout beans as a good standby. (See recipe Annex 5.)

In the case of a storm, if families have citrus fruits which were blown off their trees, they should make the best use of them. They should gather up those which are not badly bruised or broken apart; wash them well and juice them. If they must add water to the drink, remember that the water should be boiled or treated with the special tablets provided by health workers to make that water safe for drinking.

A little citrus juice in their favourite corned meat dish gives a lift to the taste, especially if the meat is slightly 'touched'. They can also save on the use of vinegar if they use citrus juice in their cooking. They can save on sugar too with orange and grapefruit juices as their beverage base. Homemade juices can be much healthier than some sold in shops and supermarkets as sugar need not be added in most cases or, if it is, the amount can be controlled.

If the family has excess fruits they should share them with others, and not allow them to go to waste. They can also share them with the various children's homes, hospitals, homes for the aged, schools and hurricane shelters.

Wheat bread may be scarce but the family may be blessed with some produce from the field — yams, bananas and plantains, for example. These are excellent bread substitutes and good old-time favourites. Boiled, roasted, baked, fried, mashed or chunky, these ground provisions go well with any meat, fish, chicken, eggs or cheese.

Take special care of the diabetic and other vulnerable groups.

The meals of these special people during an emergency are very important because food that is tasty as well as nourishing will keep the spirits high. Children, the aged and the infirm are likely to be disturbed by any sort of change from normal conditions. Pregnant women and nursing mothers have their special food needs, so do infants and children under five years old.

If the family has a diabetic member in the home, they should remember: people with diabetes have to be very careful about what they eat; but they can make tentative substitutes according to what is available. For example, if vegetables are in short supply use a serving of staple or legume in place of 2 servings of vegetable. If fruits are plentiful, substitute 3 servings of fruit for 2 staples. A diabetic must try to eat the **same amount** of food at the **same time** each day. Whatever happens, a diabetic should not starve himself. It is just as bad to eat too little as to eat too much, especially if the diabetic is on insulin.

Insulin keeps well at room temperature. If it gets cloudy when it should be clear, it is best not to use it as it may be going bad.

People with diabetes must be very careful not to get cuts or skin infections during times of stress. Their body resistance to disease and injury is generally lower than in other folk. Their skin infection or injury may take longer to heal and must be kept clean and carefully dressed.

You may have to help families:
● Prepare high energy liquid feeds for young children and some elderly persons. A concentrated liquid may be prepared consisting of: (a) a mixture of 6 parts skimmed milk powder, 2 parts oil, 1 part sugar, (b) 1 can sweetened condensed milk and 1 oz skimmed milk powder, ½ can water. Use one part of the concentrate in 4 parts water, e.g. 1 cup in 4 cups water.
● Keep a close watch on food supplies.

- Get extra food to come into the community.
- Get special foods.
- Use what they have to get the maximum, e.g. encourage breastfeeding mothers to continue to breastfeed.
- Arrange for emergency shelter.
- Follow the instructions of the health authorities.
- Get immunized if necessary.
- Give first aid.
- Prevent disease by handling garbage and human waste properly.

Annexes

ANNEX 1

SOME WORDS/TERMS USED AND THEIR MEANING

Absorption   The process by which nourishing substances pass into the blood stream after digestion.

Amputated   Cut off, e.g. limbs with spreading infections in some diabetics.

Anaemia   The name given to the condition which occurs when the blood cannot carry oxygen to all parts of the body. Persons who have anaemia usually feel weak and tired and may get infections often. Anaemia is caused by a lack of iron and certain vitamins in the diet as well as by blood loss. Anaemia is also known as thin blood.

Artery   Blood vessel which carries pure or oxygenated blood.

Atherosclerosis   The name of the disease when an artery hardens. The passage through which blood flows becomes narrow and the artery loses its elasticity.

Bagasse   Dried, crushed sugarcane fibre.

Balanced diet   Combining foods from different food groups for good nutrition.

Biogas   A type of fuel (gas) produced from animal or vegetable wastes.

Blanch   Place in boiling water for a short time (1-2 minutes).

Blood pressure   The force of the blood against the walls of the blood vessels.

By-product   Anything produced in the course of making something else. For example, molasses is a by-product of sugar.

Caesarean section — An operation during which a baby is removed from its mother by an opening in her womb.

Caliper — An instrument for measuring something round.

Carbohydrate — Nutrient group which includes sugars and starches.

Cholesterol — Fat-like substance found only in animal sources of food e.g. butter, eggs.

Colostrum — Thin, yellowish fluid which comes from the breasts from about the seventh month of pregnancy and immediately after birth until about three days after.

Concentrated — Made stronger by removing the water: for example, in dried beans the nourishment becomes more (concentrated) than in the green peas because the water has dried out.

Contraception — Preventing pregnancy through use of family planning methods.

Creche — A day nursery or day-care centre.

Dehydration — Loss of water and salts from the body, usually during diarrhoea.

Diabetes — A disease in which there is excess sugar (glucose) in the blood. There is excess sugar because sugar from digested food cannot get into the body cells as it should. Sugar cannot get to the cells because there is either not enough insulin or the body cannot use the insulin present effectively.

Digested — When food is broken down in the body into simple substances which go into the blood stream and nourish the body.

Enrichment — Replacing the nutrients which have been removed from grain during processing (milling).

Entrails   The inner organs of animals — e.g. tripe, stomach intestines.

Episode   An event which is part of a sequence.

Family pot   Foods provided or cooked for the whole family.

Feedback   Information received by a communicator in response to messages sent.

Fibre   A group of chemical substances found in the cell walls of plants. They are very important in the diet for helping to maintain good health.

Folate   One of the B vitamins.

Fortified   When a vitamin or mineral is added to make a food more nourishing: for example wheat flour is fortified with iron and B vitamins.

Gout   A disease with inflammation of the joints, especially of the big toe.

Heart attack   Sudden heart failure.

Hernia   The projection or protrusion of a part of an organ through a membrane, especially that of the abdomen or belly.

Haemoglobin   A substance in the blood containing iron which allows oxygen to be carried throughout the body.

Health Committee   A group of people in a community who meet to discuss health problems. The plan and carry out activities to correct the problems, check on progress and evaluate what has been done. A Health Committee may operate at the community, regional, national or international levels.

Homogenized   When the fat in milk is so finely divided that the cream does not separate. Goat's milk is naturally homogenized. Other kinds of milk are homogenized by processing.

Hygiene/
sanitation
Cleanliness and healthy habits.

Immunization
Protection against infectious diseases.

Insulin
A hormone (chemical messenger) produced by the pancreas which removes excess sugar from the blood into the cells.

Malnutrition
A disease caused when a person does not eat enough food or the wrong kinds of food.

Metabolism
The process by which food is built up into living things or used to supply energy in living things.

Multimix
principle
Combining foods from different food groups for good nutrition.

Nutrients
Nourishing substances in foods, e.g. proteins, minerals, vitamins, carbohydrates.

Oedema
Build up of fluid in the body, usually shown by swollen ankles.

Pasteurized
When a liquid or solid food is heated to a certain temperature for a short period of time to destroy harmful germs (bacteria).

Primary
Health Care
A concept which highlights the fact that health care is the responsibility not only of the government, but also of the community and the individual. It is based on 3 major principles:
1. Individuals and communities can be taught to take care of simple illnesses; they should have access to basic health services within the community and to more specialized care if necessary.
2. Sectors such as health, education, agriculture and community development co-operate with each other to provide food and other basic services.
3. Each individual should have responsibility for his own health care and that of others in the community.

Rehydration   Replacing water and salts by means of fluids and/or the oral rehydration solution.

Solar drier   Special type of oven or 'hot box' heated by the sun and used for drying foods or other produce.

Solution   A mixture which is produced when a solid such as sugar dissolves (mixes) in a liquid, for example water.

Surveillance   (Pronounced "sur-vey-ance") keeping watch, usually over a person's or community's general health and nutrition.

Sphygmo-manometer   The instrument used to measure blood pressure.

Stroke   Sudden inability to feel and move, because of blockage or rupture of an artery (blood vessel) in the brain.

Symptom   A sign that something is happening to the body or to the way in which the body functions, which is different from normal. It shows that disease or injury is present.

Tonic   Usually a drink which is supposed to be nourishing — may be bought or home-made.

Toto   A quick bread (see selected recipes, Annex 7).

Vegetarian   (a) A diet which does not contain meat or any other animal products; apart from dairy products and eggs.
    (b) A person who does not eat meat or any animal products; apart from dairy products and eggs.

ANNEX 2
SOME UNITS OF METRIC MEASUREMENT

Weight

1000 kilograms	=	1 metric ton (tonne)

Kilogram (shortened kg)
or

1000 grams (shortened g)	=	a little more than 2 pounds (2.2 or $2\frac{1}{5}$ lbs)
500 grams	=	a little more than 1 pound (1.1 or $1\frac{1}{10}$ lbs)
454 grams	=	1 pound
250 grams	=	a little more than $\frac{1}{2}$ pound (9 oz)
100 grams	=	a little less than $\frac{1}{4}$ pound ($3\frac{1}{2}$ oz)
28.4 grams	=	1 oz
1 gram	=	0.035 oz

Capacity

Litre (shortened L) = a little more than 1 US quart or 32 oz (35 oz)

or

1000 millilitres (shortened mL) = or
a little less than 1 imperial quart or 40 oz (35 oz) or 0.22 imperial gallons

Volume

Cubic centimetres (shortened cc)*

500 cc	=	2 measuring cups or 500 grams
250 cc	=	1 measuring cup or 250 grams
125 cc	=	½ measuring cup or 125 grams
60 cc	=	¼ measuring cup or 60 grams
15 cc	=	1 tablespoon or 15 grams
5 cc	=	1 teaspoon or 5 grams

These gram weights for a given volume are for most solids and liquids such as sugar, rice, butter, water and fluid milk. Powdered or flaky items such as flour, skimmed milk powder and oats would weigh less, that is, 140 grams per cup or 3½ cups per pound. One cup of cooking oil weighs about 200 grams. So oil is lighter than water.

Length

1.6 kilometres	=	1 mile
1 kilometre (shortened km)		
or	=	0.6 mile
1,000 metres (shortened m)		
1 metre	=	a little more than 1 yard (1.09 yards or 39 inches)
30.5 centimetres (cm)	=	1 foot
2.5 centimetres (cm)		
or	=	1 inch
25.4 millimetres (mm)		

Area

10,000 square metres (sq.m)	=	1 hectare
0.42 hectares (ha)	=	1 acre

Temperature

1°F = 5/9°C
100°F = 56°C
200°F = 111°C
300°F = 167°C
350°F = 193°C
400°F = 222°C
450°F = 250°C

ANNEX 3

COPING WITH DISASTERS

In times of disaster such as after hurricanes, storms, floods, earthquakes and fires, people in the community may need special attention. They may need food, clothes, shelter, medical and nursing care and other help urgently. Safe drinking water and food may become scarce. Poor sanitation may increase rats, flies and other disease carriers. Many people may be at risk of infections, disease and malnutrition.

The community worker can:

1. Help people to use available food, particularly those which have fallen off trees and may go to waste.
2. Advise people to get into each meal a staple, some fat and some food from animals.
3. Keep a close watch on food supplies.

4. Arrange for extra food to come into the community.
5. See to it that special foods go to those for whom they are intended.
6. Encourage breastfeeding mothers to continue to breastfeed.
7. Arrange for emergency shelter and feeding of people who have lost their homes.
8. Prepare high energy liquid feeds for young children and some elderly persons. A concentrated liquid may be prepared consisting of: (a) a mixture of 6 parts skimmed milk powder, 2 parts oil, 1 part sugar, (b) 1 can sweetened condensed milk and 1 tablespoon skimmed milk powder, ½ can water. Use one part of the concentrate in 4 parts water for example 1 cup in 4 cups water.
9. Encourage people to drink only water or other liquids which they know are safe.
10. Show people how to make and keep water safe by boiling for 10-15 minutes. If boiling is difficult, 1 drop of bleach may be added to each litre of clear water or 3 drops to cloudy water. Stir and allow the water to stand for 30 minutes before drinking. If the water does not taste or smell too strongly of chlorine add a few more drops of bleach. Wait for 15 minutes and taste again.
11. Help people to follow the instructions of the health authorities.
12. See to it that people are immunized if necessary.
13. Give first aid.
14. Show people how to handle garbage and human waste to prevent disease.

ANNEX 4

IDEAS ON HOW TO SAVE FUEL ENERGY IN FOOD PREPARATION*

1. If you use wood or charcoal to cook on, find out about improved stoves or 'jikos' which burn less fuel.
2. Do not keep the pilot light on a gas cooker going all the time. Turn it off and use matches to light burners when needed.
3. Use the right size pot for a gas or kerosene (parafin) burner. A small pot on a large burner wastes energy.
4. Put the pot on the burner before turning on the flame.
5. Use a low flame for cooking. High flames which give a rolling boil waste food and fuel.

*(Adapted from: Scientific Research Council, Jamaica)

6. Keep the lid on the pot — steam builds up and helps to cook foods quicker.
7. Cook several items at the same time using a double or triple boiler. Improvise your own double or triple boiler or steamers by using pots or dishes of varying sizes over one another, or a colander sieve in a pot.
8. Turn off flame just before foods are cooked and keep pot covered. The heat left in the pot will finish the cooking.
9. Cook foods only until tender.
10. Cook for all household members at one time.
11. Cut foods in small pieces so that they will cook quickly.
12. Cook in the smallest amount of liquid possible. It takes more energy to heat up large amounts of liquid. In cooking spinach for example, the water left clinging to the leaves is adequate.
13. Don't brown meats by high temperature. This toughens the meat and makes it take longer to cook.
14. If you tenderize tough meats before cooking, they will cook quicker. Here's how:
    — Wrap meat in pawpaw leaves or include a chopped young pawpaw in the seasoning.
    N.B. The substance in the pawpaw which tenderizes is destroyed by heat. Add the young pawpaw to the meat before it is heated.
    — chop or beat meat to break up fibres.
15. Soak dried beans before cooking. Do not use baking soda to tenderize them. Soda destroys the B vitamins in beans.
16. Use the right size pot to suit the amount of food being prepared. It is a waste of energy to fry one egg in a large frying pan in which four could have been done at the same time.
17. Make good use of the pressure cooker if you have one. Items like dried peas, trotters, or tripe cook much quicker than in an ordinary pot.

ANNEX 5

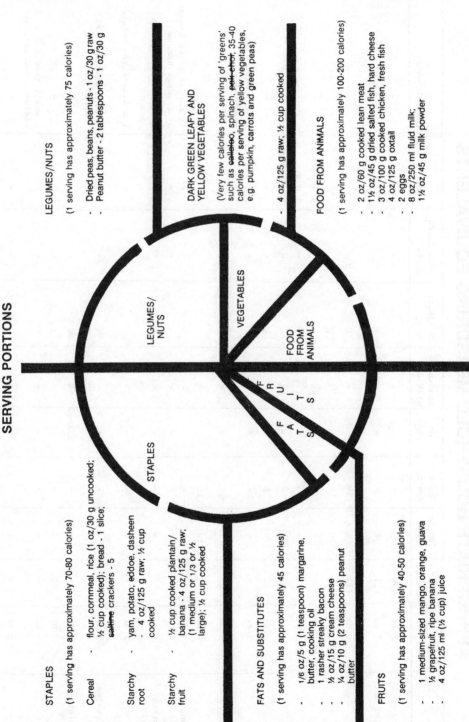

SERVING PORTIONS

STAPLES

(1 serving has approximately 70-80 calories)

Cereal - flour, cornmeal, rice (1 oz/30 g uncooked; ½ cup cooked); bread - 1 slice; saline crackers - 5

Starchy root - yam, potato, eddoe, dasheen - 4 oz/125 g raw; ½ cup cooked

Starchy fruit - ½ cup cooked plantain/banana - 4 oz/125 g raw; (1 medium or 1/3 or ½ large); ½ cup cooked

FATS AND SUBSTITUTES

(1 serving has approximately 45 calories)

- 1/6 oz/5 g (1 teaspoon) margarine, butter, cooking oil
- 1 rasher streaky bacon
- ½ oz/15 g cream cheese
- ¼ oz/10 g (2 teaspoons) peanut butter

FRUITS

(1 serving has approximately 40-50 calories)

- 1 medium-sized mango, orange, guava
- ½ grapefruit, ripe banana
- 4 oz/125 ml (½ cup) juice

LEGUMES/NUTS

(1 serving has approximately 75 calories)

- Dried peas, beans, peanuts - 1 oz/30 g raw
- Peanut butter - 2 tablespoons - 1 oz/30 g

DARK GREEN LEAFY AND YELLOW VEGETABLES

(Very few calories per serving of 'greens' such as calaloo, spinach, pak-choi, 35-40 calories per serving of yellow vegetables, e.g. pumpkin, carrots and green peas)

- 4 oz/125 g raw; ½ cup cooked

FOOD FROM ANIMALS

(1 serving has approximately 100-200 calories)

- 2 oz/60 g cooked lean meat
- 1½ oz/45 g dried salted fish, hard cheese
- 3 oz/100 g cooked chicken, fresh fish
- 4 oz/125 g oxtail
- 2 eggs
- 8 oz/250 ml fluid milk;
  1½ oz/45 g milk powder

STAPLES

LEGUMES/NUTS

VEGETABLES

FOOD FROM ANIMALS

FRUITS

FATS

ANNEX 6

APPROPRIATE HOUSEHOLD MEASURING EQUIVALENTS

	Weights	Tea-spoon	Table-spoon	Dessert spoon	Cook spoon	Condensed milk can	Drinking cup	6-oz Juice glass	Pint	Crude Measure
Condensed milk	2 oz	9	3	-	-	-	-	-	-	-
Evaporated milk	2 oz	12	4	-	-	-	¼	1/3	-	-
Skimmed milk powder	1 oz	12	4	5½	-	-	¼	1/3	-	-
Water *	4 fl. oz	-	10	12	-	1/3	¾	¾	-	-
Water	20 fl. oz	-	-	-	-	2½	-	-	1 Imperial	-
Water	16 fl. oz	-	-	-	-	1¾	-	-	1 U.S.	-
Water	10 fl. oz	-	-	-	-	1¼	-	-	½ Imperial	-
Rice	2 oz	12	4	5	2	-	¼	-	-	-
Plantain	3 oz	-	-	-	-	-	-	-	-	½ of a medium-sized plantain
Cornmeal	2 oz	21	7	10	4	½	½	½	-	-
Oats	2 oz	-	10	10	5	½	-	-	-	-
Green banana	3 oz	-	-	-	-	-	-	-	-	1½ medium-sized banana
(peeled)	3 oz	-	-	-	-	-	-	-	-	or 1 large banana
Sweet potato (peeled)	3 oz	-	-	-	-	-	-	-	-	½ of a medium-sized potato
Potato (peeled)	3 oz	-	-		-	-	-	-	-	1 medium-sized potato
Carrot (peeled)	1 oz			-		-	-	-	-	½ of a medium-sized carrot
Red peas/kidney beans	2 oz	-	-	-	1 heaped	¼	¼	-	-	-
Sugar D	1 oz	9¼	3	4	-	-	-	-	-	-
Sardine	1 oz	-	-	-	-	-	-	-	-	3 small sardines or 2 medium-sized sardines
Margarine	½ oz	3	1	-	-	-	-	-	-	-

*Cow's and reconstituted skimmed milk as for water.

ANNEX 7

SELECTED RECIPES

Corning/pickling meat

The meats which are usually corned or pickled are pork and beef. Meat can be corned or pickled by a dry or wet method.

Wet pickle for 10-15 lbs (5-7 kilos) meat

0.75 kilo	1½ lbs	salt
0.25 kilos	½ lb	brown sugar
5.0 grams	½ tbsp	ground allspice (pimento)
2.0 grams	½ tsp	powdered cloves
25 grams	1½ tbsp	saltpetre
6 litres	1½ gallons	water

Put all the pickle ingredients into a large, clean pot; bring to boiling point and boil for 10-15 minutes. Skim, strain and use when cold. Clean meat with a rag dipped in vinegar and gash or score all over. Place in a plastic pail or earthenware pot or bowl. Cover the meat entirely with the liquid brine and cover the container tightly. If pickle does not fully cover meat, turn daily so all sides will be evenly soaked. Keep in pickle for 2-3 weeks or remove pieces as needed.

When ready to use, rinse the meat thoroughly, soak overnight or for at least two hours and boil in fresh water or prepare in other ways.

Dry pickle for about 10-15 lbs (5-7 kilos) meat

1 kilo	2 lbs	salt
½ kilo	1lb	brown sugar
2 grams	½ tsp	powdered ginger
2 grams	½ tsp	ground cloves
25 grams	1½ tbsp	saltpetre
20 grams	2 tbsp	ground black pepper
5 grams	½ tbsp	ground allspice (pimento)

Wipe meat with cloth dipped in vinegar, then pat dry with paper or towel. Rub meat all over with about half of the salt and leave for twelve to fourteen hours in covered plastic pail or earthenware bowl. Mix the remaining salt and all the other ingredients and rub the meat daily with a part for a week until sufficiently spiced.

When ready to use, wash and soak the meat overnight or for at least two hours, drain and prepare in your favourite way.

Variation

Omit the powdered spices and substitute dried cinnamon, pimento or bay leaves broken into fine pieces, chopped hot pepper, garlic and thyme and whole pimento berries. Mix these with the salt and sugar and rub into meat thoroughly. Leave in covered pail or bowl for one to two weeks, turning meat occasionally.

> **Note: If it is possible to refrigerate the meat while it is in the pickle or brine, use only half as much salt and sugar.**

SPROUTING BEANS

Beans can be sprouted in a wide mouth jar, cloth bag, or clean flower pot, as long as there is some provision for draining off excess water.

The container should be large enough for the beans to swell to 3-4 times their original bulk. Soya or mung beans are usually sprouted but a range of edible peas and beans can be used.

A. Preparing the sprouting vessel

Different kinds of sprouting vessels may be used:

(a) Flower pot — An unglazed earthenware (clay) pot is best. Put a clean wire netting or cloth across the hole in the bottom. Add soaked beans. Cover the pot with a damp cloth and cardboard and raise slightly so all the water drains out after watering the beans.

(b) Jar — Cover the mouth of an ordinary jam jar with a piece of clean, fine mesh wire or cloth, after putting in the soaked beans. Turn the jar upside down in a dark, cool place.

(c) Cloth bag — Suspend the cloth bag with the soaked beans in a pan, with a little water in the bottom. The beans should not touch the water.

B. Preparing the beans

Soak beans overnight — 1 part beans to 3 parts water. In the morning, drain beans and put them in the sprouting vessel. Cover and leave in a warm, dark place. Flood with lukewarm water, 3-4 times during the first day.

After the second day the beans get warm so you may need to sprinkle them with cool water or place ice cubes in the container during the last day. In 2-3 days the sprouts will be 2-3 inches tall.

Keep sprouts in a cool place like any other vegetable. Better still, use immediately, or blanch for 2-3 minutes and freeze.

C. How to use sprouted beans

Use sprouts with beans attached. Add cooked sprouts to vegetable combinations, soups, stews, casseroles, scrambled eggs, omelettes, cook-ups, salted and pickled fish. Stir-fry or cook lightly and serve as a plain vegetable.

To lightly cook sprouts, place one or two teaspoons of cooking oil or margarine in a frying pan. Add 1-2 tablespoons chopped onion. Add 1-2 cups sprouts, $\frac{1}{4}$ cup water and other desired seasoning such as soy sauce. Cover and cook for 5-8 minutes.

Steam sprouts for 4-5 minutes and stir-fry in a small amount of oil. The cooked sprouts should be chewy but crisp.

MAKING PRESERVES

Jams, jellies, marmalade, chutneys and pickles are common preserves found in many homes. **Jams** contain the whole fruit or fruit pulp, whereas **jellies** are made from the juice filtered off from the boiled fruit. Using sugar and cooking at high temperatures for long periods will preserve the fruit from spoiling. In the case of chutneys and pickles, vinegar adds extra protection. Because of the long heating process, these preserves do not have high nutritive value in terms of their Vitamin C (ascorbic acid) content. So guava jelly or jam is not a good source of Vitamin C, although fresh guavas are an excellent source.

HOW TO MAKE JAMS AND JELLIES

● To produce a good jam or jelly, use the exact amount of sugar to fruit indicated, also the right proportion of sugar, acid, pectin or other jelling substance. Fruits contain different amounts of acid and pectin. So fruits that are rich in both acid and pectin, such as guava, are easy to gel. Some fruits are rich in pectin and low in acid. The reverse is also true, as in pawpaw and pineapple, so it's a good idea to combine fruits and juices when making preserves, to get the right balance of acid and pectin. You could also combine slightly under-ripe fruits (which have a higher pectin content than ripe fruits) with fully ripened, full-flavoured fruit. When a fruit has little natural pectin, you'll need to add more fruit than sugar. Also, add a little acid in the form of lemon or lime juice or commercial pectin. When a fruit is rich in pectin, add more sugar than fruit. In general, use 1 cup fruit or juice to 1 cup sugar.

- Use fresh, sound and ripe fruits. You may also add slightly under-ripe fruits to produce more natural pectin. Wash fruits well before using and remove bad spots and ends.
- Stew fruits slowly to extract pectin, soften skin and give a good colour to the finished jam or jelly.
- Place the stewed fruit in a bag to filter the juice for jelly-making. Do not squeeze the bag as the jelly will be cloudy instead of clear.
- It's best to use a large pot so that there will be plenty of space for the jam or jelly to boil vigorously without splashing or boiling over.
- Place the sugar and fruit pulp or juice in the pan and stir the mixture until the sugar dissolves. Boil rapidly without further stirring.
- Early in the process, test for jelling or setting. Some jams are ready within 3-5 minutes, others take 10-15 minutes or more after boiling begins. Many fruits lose their setting qualities if boiled too long. To test for jelling, place a little of the boiling mixture on a saucer and allow to cool. Tilt the saucer. If the mixture runs off it is not yet done; if it stands firm, it is done.

MAKING YOUR OWN VINEGAR

Vinegar is made through a natural process called fermentation. In this process, moulds, yeast and other living organisms (which we cannot see) feed on sugars and starches and produce acid and alcohol. The acid product is **vinegar** and the alcohol product is **wine**. Wine making requires a lot of care.

Vinegar can be made from the juices and syrup of sugar-cane, fruits and cocoa beans. Here's how to make your own:

Put the freshly extracted juices in a clean jar or other glass or pottery container. Cover loosely and leave for several months. Strain off the clear portion. Bottle in clean, sterilized bottles. Stopper tightly and leave to age. The acid will keep the vinegar safe for years. Making vinegar from fruit juices or cane liquor is a way of preserving a product that might otherwise be wasted.

FREEZING

Freezing retards the growth of tiny creatures which cause food to spoil, is convenient and helps to retain natural flavour, texture, colour and nutritive value much better than any other methods commonly used.

Frozen foods can save time and money and add interest and variety to meals. Some foods which freeze well are green peas, carrots, pumpkin and cabbage (cut into neat pieces), fruits, juices and strained vegetables.

Tips for freezing
— Sort foods according to stage of maturity, if possible.
— Wash well, peel (if necessary) and cut into pieces of desired size.
— Blanch or scald vegetables.
— Cool quickly in ice-cold water.
— Drain thoroughly before packaging.
— Pack in air-tight bags, boxes or tubs.
— Place fruits in a medium sugar syrup* or add sugar directly to fruit.

A medium sugar syrup is made by adding 500 g (1 lb) sugar (preferably white, granulated) to 1 litre (quart) water, stirring and boiling for 5-6 minutes or 1 minute after the mixture begins to boil.

FLOURS FROM PROVISIONS

Making flour is one way in which we can preserve and store provisions when supplies are plentiful.

To make flour
1. Peel and wash the provision in clean water. (Add lime juice to the water to prevent darkening of the provision.)
2. Slice very thinly.
3. Place the thin slices on a clean tray or wire rack.
4. Put the tray in the sun or in a solar drier or a slow oven and dry the slices until crisp.
5. Grind or pound the dried provisions, then sift.
6. Store the flour in a clean, dry container. Cover it tightly.

The amount of provision flour you use with the wheat flour will depend on your taste. Generally, a mixture of one part (e.g. 1 cup) of provision flour and 2 parts of wheat flour makes very good products. Use ½ cup banana flour to 2 cups wheat flour for tasty products with an attractive colour.

When you use these flours with wheat flour to make home-made breads, you'll need to add a bit more liquid than you would use for wheat flour alone. This will make the finished product moist.

CORNED PORK CURRY

½ lb boiled lean corned pork
3 tbsp cooking oil
4 medium-sized spinach leaves

1 large onion, chopped
2 tsp curry powder
½ cup warm water
1 clove garlic, chopped

1. Cut boiled pork into bite-sized pieces.
2. Heat oil in a pot. Add corned pork and toss until lightly browned.
3. Add spinach, seasoning and warm water.
4. Cover and simmer for 5-10 minutes. Serve hot with fluffy rice.

[**Makes 3-4 servings.**]

CORNED PORK AND CABBAGE

½ lb corned pork
½ lb cabbage, shredded or
4 medium-sized spinach leaves
1 large onion sliced

¼ hot pepper chopped or
¼ tsp black pepper
2 tbsp ketchup
2 tbsp cooking oil
1 quart water

1. Rinse pork, soak for about two hours and boil in water until tender.
2. Drain, cook and cut into small pieces.
3. Heat oil in frying pan and fry pork until lightly brown.
4. Add cabbage and seasoning. Toss for 5-10 minutes.
Serve with rice or green bananas or meal dumplings.

[**Makes 3-4 servings.**]

FLUFFY FISH FRITTER

1 (3½ oz) can sardines or
   mackerel
1½ cups flour
1½ tsp baking powder
1 medium onion, chopped
Oil for frying

¼ tsp black pepper or hot pepper
1 tsp vinegar or lime juice
¼ tsp salt
1 egg, well beaten
¾-1 cup water

1. Combine canned fish (mashed with a fork) with dry ingredients, seasoning and beaten egg.
2. Add water and mix to a soft batter.
3. Drop by dessert spoon into hot fat. Turn once.
4. Drain on absorbent paper.
Serve with a hot or cold beverage and a ripe banana for breakfast, lunch or supper.

[**Makes 16-18 fritters.**]

FISH/BANANA MEDLEY

½ lb salted fish or
2 (3½ oz) cans sardine or
 mackerel
1 large dry coconut
1 quart warm water
1 oz salt pork (optional)
6 pimento seeds (allspice)

12 fingers green bananas (figs)
1 large onion
1 whole hot pepper
2 cloves garlic, chopped
1 sprig thyme
1 tsp curry powder

1. Soak salted fish for one hour and flake.
2. Grate coconut and extract 'milk' with warm water.
3. Place milk in pot and boil.
4. Add chopped pork, curry powder and pimento seeds.
5. Peel, wash and cut bananas in halves and add to pot along with flaked salted fish.
6. Cook for 20 minutes.

[**Makes 4 servings.**]
If canned fish is used, add after cooking bananas for 20 minutes. Add seasoning and cook until liquid is thick and flavours are well blended.

Variation
Substitute banana or plantain dumplings for bananas. To make dumplings:
1. Peel, wash and grate 3 or 4 large fingers of green bananas or 1 large green plantain.
2. Add 1 cup or more of flour.
3. Mix until dough comes together in a ball.
4. Roll out into a log and cut into small even pieces or break off small pieces of dough and make round dumplings.
Note: The grated plantain or banana is moist so there is no need to add water. Grated sweet cassava or yam can be substituted for green bananas or plantains.

SCRAMBLED EGGS WITH BEAN SPROUTS

1 cup finely chopped onion
½ tsp salt
1-2 tbsp cooking oil
4 eggs, slightly beaten
2 cups raw bean sprouts

1. Add onion and salt to slightly beaten eggs. Let stand 5-10 minutes.
2. Stir-fry bean sprouts 5 minutes in frying pan with hot oil.
3. Add egg mixture and stir.
4. Cook until eggs are well scrambled. Serve over plain rice.

[**Makes 4 servings.**]

GREEN PLANTAIN PANCAKE

1 green plantain   1 medium onion, chopped finely
¼ tsp salt   ¼ medium-sized sweet pepper,
1 egg, beaten   chopped finely

1. Peel and shred plantain.
2. Combine with other ingredients, mixing well.
3. Drop by heaped tablespoon on a hot, generously greased frying pan or griddle.
4. Flatten with lifter and fry for 3 minutes on each side.
5. Remove from pan/griddle and serve hot with roast pork or other meat of choice.

[**Makes 3-4 servings.**]

SPICED BAKED PLANTAIN

1 ripe plantain   ⅛ tsp cinnamon or mixed spice
2 tbsp melted margarine   ¼ tsp ground ginger
1 tbsp sugar

1. Remove skin and cut plantain crosswise in four.
2. Place in greased baking dish.
3. Brush with margarine and sprinkle with sugar, ginger and cinnamon.
4. Bake at 350°F for 15 minutes until lightly browned.
Serve with meat of choice.

[**Makes 4 servings.**]

DUCKUNOO

1 lb cornmeal   1 tsp cinnamon
1 cup grated yam   ½ lb sugar
½ cup grated coconut   1 tbsp molasses

½ cup dried fruits (optional)   2 tsp vanilla
1 tsp mixed spice   2½ cups coconut 'milk' or cow's
                                    milk

1. Have ready, large pot of boiling, spiced water, pieces of quailed (passed over fire or boiling water) green banana leaf or squares of foil and banana bark or twine.
2. Mix together cornmeal, grated yam, sugar, grated coconut, fruits and spices.
3. Add cow's milk or coconut 'milk', molasses and vanilla, stirring well.
4. Place ½ cup to 1 cup of the mixture on pieces of quailed banana leaf or aluminium foil. Make a parcel and tie with twine or dried banana bark.
5. Cook the parcels in boiling water to cover, for about 40 minutes. Serve for breakfast, lunch or supper with vegetables and fruit juice. It's a good item to pack in the lunch box too!

[**Makes 4-6 servings.**]

QUICK SPICED BUN

1 cup provision flour   ¼ cup melted margarine
2 cups wheat flour   1 tbs vanilla
2 tsp baking powder   2 tbs molasses (optional)
2 tsp mixed spice   1 cup brown sugar
¼ tsp ground, dried orange   1 egg, well beaten
   peel (optional)   1 cup milk
1 tsp aniseed

1. Heat oven to 300°F.
2. Mix together flours, baking powder and spices in a bowl.
3. Heat* molasses and combine with sugar, milk, beaten egg, margarine and vanilla.
4. Add liquid mixture to dry ingredients, stirring lightly.
5. Pour into greased 2 lb loaf pan and bake in oven for 40-50 minutes.

Heating makes the molasses mix easily with the other ingredients.

6. Remove from oven. Brush with syrup if desired and let sit for a day before eating.

[**Makes a 2 lb loaf 6-8 servings.**]

Variation 1: 'TOTO' (a Jamaican recipe)
Omit: aniseed
Add: 1 tsp baking soda and
½ cups grated coconut

Bake in a square pan at a slightly higher temperature (350°F) for 30-40 minutes.

[**Makes 12 servings.**]

Variation 2: 'BULLA' (another Jamaican recipe)
Omit: aniseed, baking powder and egg
Add: ½ cup sugar
3 tsp baking soda
½ tsp ground ginger

1. After mixing dry and liquid ingredients, let mixture sit for 10-15 minutes.
2. Place on well-floured board and knead.
3. Roll out about ¼ inches thick and cut out circles about 3 inches wide.
4. Place circles on a greased baking sheet and bake at 350°F for 20 minutes.

Serve these quick breads with cheese and milk for snacks, lunch or supper.

[**Makes 20 bullas.**]

ANNEX 8
USEFUL REFERENCES

Books

1. *Helping Mothers To Breast Feed* F. Savage-King AMREF P.O.B 30125, Nairobi.
2. *Nutrition For Developing Countries:* King, Morley and Burgess — Written in simple English, with exercises which can be undertaken in the community (ELBS edition)
3. *Nutrition And Families:* Jean Richie — A well illustrated and practical book for those working in nutrition and family health, particularly in Africa.
4. *Manual On Feeding Infants And Young Children:* Cameron and Hofvander — A new edition completely re-written, simple and practical. O.U.P.
5. *Child-To-Child:* Prepared for the International Year of the Child, this describes how older children can help younger children's health and development. Also free Newsletter and activity sheets.

6. *Breast Feeding In Practice:* E. Helsing and F. Savage King — An aid to health workers to guide and support mothers in successful breast feeding. Also in Spanish.

7. *Breast Feeding, The Biological Option:* G.J. Ebrahim. (ELBS editions available only while stocks last).

8. *Nutrition In Mother And Child Health:* G.J. Ebrahim — Intended mainly for nutritionalists and health personnel involved in running district level services.

9. *Practising Health For All:* D. Morley, J. Rohde, G. Williams — Articles from seventeen countries describing primary health care successes and problems. Essential reading for those who think that health care is a right and duty for all.

10. *State Of The Worlds Children:* UNICEF — 1984 edition describes their priorities towards GOBI 1985 edition will be supplied from about February onwards.

11. *Rural Development; Putting The Last First:* Robert Chambers — Describes why we all fail to reach the very poor and those who need help most.

12. *Community Health:* edited by C.H. Wood, J.P. Vaughan and H. de Glanville — written to help health workers extend their thoughts to the health of the community as a whole.

13. *Happy Health Children.* Hampton, (TALC Macmillan)

14. *Better Child Care.* Tregoning, (TALC. Macmillan)

15. *Primary Child Care:* King, Maurice and others. Book One. A manual for Health Workers. Oxford, Oxford University Press, 1978.

16. *See How They Grow* David, Morley and Margaret Woodland. — Monitoring Child Growth for Appropriate Health Care in Developing Countries. New York, Oxford University Press, 1979.

17. *Where there is no doctor,* David, Werner. Palo Alto, California, Hesperian Foundation, 1977.

18. *Helping Health Workers Learn.* David, Werner and Bill Bower. Palo Alto, California. Hesperian Foundation, 1982.

Accessories

19. *'Road To Health' Weight Charts:* Growth charts of this type are now widely used. The TALC chart has undergone extensive testing and development over 20 years. We strongly advise gaining experience with these before developing your own modifications. Available in English, Arabic, French, Portuguese or Spanish. A sample chart will be sent free on request.

20. *Flannelgraph of the 'Road To Health' Chart:* The introduction of growth charts is not easy. Many health workers are unused to the

concept involved in completing a growth curve. Even more have problems in fully understanding and interpreting a growth curve. Exercises in which they are involved using a flannelgraph can be an important step in the successful use of growth charts. The flannelgraph consists of a growth chart printed on cloth 91 cm x 62 cm. Two sheets of symbols to cut out. Complete with sheets describing the exercises in detail.

21. *Nutrition And Child Health Flannelgraph:* This flannelgraph is appropriate for village teaching in large areas of Africa. There are seven sheets of cutouts and detailed illustrated instructions. The subjects covered are:

Feed your children often
Give your child plenty of soup
Learning to eat
Diarrhoea prevention and home management
Measles
Come to the Child Welfare Clinic

A very useful aid for those involved in teaching nutrition, health and development at village level. Portuguese text available.

22. *Weight For Height Chart:* The weight for height chart is a new technique to simplify the measurements of children's nutrition. It may be used in conjunction with a Road to Health chart or independently, if weighings are infrequent, or if the age of the child is not know.

23. *Echeverri Tape:* A new idea for measuring and recording upper arm circumference from 0-6 years. Kits consist of 20 charts, 1 tape with cursor and an instruction sheet. Sample chart and tape free on request.

24. *Set Of Four Measuring Spoons:* Scoops for clinic use. Measure appropriate quantities of glucose and salts for a litre of rehydration fluid.

25. *Sugar And Salt Measures:* Spoons for home use, to prevent dehydration (English, Arabic, Chinese, French, Portuguese, Spanish) Special rates for order over 500.

For information on charts, low cost, scales, sets of slides and any of these books write to:-

TALC
Box 49
St. Albans
Hertfordshire   AL1 4AX
United Kingdom

INDEX